Vietnam War Nurses
at the Ready

D1551329

ALSO EDITED BY PATRICIA RUSHTON

*Vietnam War Nurses: Personal Accounts
of 18 Americans* (McFarland, 2013)

*Gulf War Nurses: Personal Accounts
of 14 Americans, 1990–1991 and 2003–2010*
(McFarland, 2011)

Vietnam War Nurses at the Ready

Seventeen Personal Accounts

Edited by PATRICIA RUSHTON

McFarland & Company, Inc., Publishers

Jefferson, North Carolina

LIBRARY OF CONGRESS CATALOGUING-IN-PUBLICATION DATA

Names: Rushton, Patricia, editor.
Title: Vietnam war nurses at the ready: seventeen personal accounts /
edited Patricia Rushton.
Description: Jefferson, North Carolina : McFarland & Company, Inc.,
Publishers, 2023 | Includes index.
Identifiers: LCCN 2022062104 | ISBN 9781476690971 (paperback : acid free paper) ∞
ISBN 9781476648828 (ebook)
Subjects: LCSH: Vietnam War, 1961–1975—Medical care. | Vietnam War,
1961–1975—Personal narratives, American. | United States. Army Nurse
Corps—Biography. | United States. Army Nurse Corps—History—Vietnam War,
1961–1975. | United States—Armed Forces—Nurses—Biography. |
Military nursing—United States—History—20th century. | Military nursing—
Vietnam—History—20th century. | BISAC: HISTORY / Wars & Conflicts /
Vietnam War | MEDICAL / Nursing / General
Classification: LCC DS559.44 .R87 2023 | DDC 959.704/37—dc23/eng/20230103
LC record available at https://lccn.loc.gov/2022062104

BRITISH LIBRARY CATALOGUING DATA ARE AVAILABLE

ISBN (print) 978-1-4766-9097-1
ISBN (ebook) 978-1-4766-4882-8

Front cover: Ensign Anne Kuhn Gartner repositioning a patient
in the medical ward; (bottom) USS *Repose* (AH 16) off the coast
of South Vietnam (U.S. Navy Medicine Historical Files)

Printed in the United States of America

*McFarland & Company, Inc., Publishers
Box 611, Jefferson, North Carolina 28640
www.mcfarlandpub.com*

Table of Contents

Preface

THE EXPERIENCES OF NURSES are not often shared with the public in general. As patients or clients, we see them function on the worst days of our lives, but their actions and contributions to public wellbeing may not enter our consciousness during our normal activities. They may share their experiences with family, friends or colleagues, but may not publicize their work.

The experiences of military nurses are almost never shared with the general public. They are infrequently shared with family or friends. They are not well known because the nurses may not be asked to share them. The experiences can be frightening and traumatizing for military nurses, have some understanding from military colleagues and be beyond the comprehension of family, friends or civilian colleagues. The nurses may feel they having nothing special to offer the profession or the public as they were "simply doing their job." However, the experiences of military nurses at war shape their lives, their interactions with others and their contributions to the nursing profession and the community in profound ways.

This is the second volume of stories told by nurses who served during the Vietnam conflict. As in the first volume, *Vietnam War Nurses: Personal Accounts of 18 Americans* (McFarland, 2013), these accounts tell the amazing experiences of nurses who served their country and the troops who defended it during the Vietnam conflict. As in the first volume, these nurses began their careers during the Vietnam Era, but continued their careers and possibly made their most important contributions in the years after that war. It was the honor of this editor to be associated with these people, to record their stories and to be one of them.

1

Phyllis Barkus

Phyllis grew up in the United States Navy Nurse Corps—
from having difficulty giving an order to being the Deputy
Director of Nursing for the Naval Inspector General

It was a fluke that I started out in nursing. I graduated from high school at 16 from Bishop McDonald Memorial High School in Brooklyn, New York, in June, 1957. I got a New York State scholarship for nursing. You had to use it in New York State. There weren't many baccalaureate programs in the fifties, none in New York, that would admit me at 16. I went to St. Catherine's Hospital in Brooklyn, New York, a three-year school of nursing.

Entering nursing school at 16, I would graduate at 19. I wouldn't be able to sit for state boards until I was 21. The law was changed before I graduated. All you had to do was graduate from an accredited school. I graduated from St. Catherine's in June 1960, about the beginning of activity in the Vietnam War. As nursing students, we did not even know about Vietnam. That was not even a consideration. A classmate always wanted to go into the Navy. She said, "Please, would you come with me to St. Albans Naval Hospital for a tour." I said, "Okay, I will go for a tour, but I'm not signing any papers." I went and it sounded good. The Navy would station us together on the buddy program for that first tour. I was commissioned an ensign in May 1961. My friend and I were stationed in Pensacola after 12 weeks of officer indoctrination in Newport, Rhode Island. Pensacola was a wonderful first duty station combining professional excellence and social activity.

Pensacola was a long way from home. I was only 20. My mother had to sign the consent form for me to go into the Navy. I was terribly homesick. I cried myself to sleep every night. That was in September 1961. They told us at Newport, "Oh yes, you'll be able to get leave for Christmas when you get to your duty station." Three of us went down to Pensacola together from Newport. We reported aboard December 7, 1961. We did not get leave for Christmas. We were living in the BOQ. It was really kind of depressing. We decorated a fan for Christmas. We said, "We'll go out and have a nice Christmas dinner." Nothing was open. We finally found a cafeteria. In the meantime, we met the people from whom we would eventually end up renting our home. They invited us to come over that evening. It was a very nice Christmas after all. I still continued to cry myself to sleep.

I was granted leave in February 1962. It was cancelled because they were having an inspector general coming for inspection. I went in April '62. When I came back, I was over the homesickness. I think I would never have left New York if I had not gone into the Navy. Before entering the Navy, I felt that there was no life outside of New York. When I returned from leave, I came back with the sense that this is a neat place to be.

We lived in the BOQ until January 1962, when we moved into a three-bedroom house. There were a lot of changes during my tour in Pensacola. I moved into a house, learned to drive, bought a car. In your youth, you don't realize all those changes going on. You don't realize all the stress that's there. It is just something that you need to do. Phone calls were very expensive. You wrote. You hung in there.

In Pensacola, I was oriented to a surgical unit. Military nursing was difficult for me. I wasn't used to telling patients to get out of bed or giving orders. You were the nurse, the caregiver. In nursing school, we had no nurse's aides at the time. You did everything. It was a little difficult to be assertive with patients and corpsmen. A lot of them were older than I was. On Fridays, we had our captain's inspections. I'm coming out of nursing school and a sheltered life. You trust everyone when they say that they have done something. Part of our responsibility was the sigmoidoscopy room. This corpsman told me that he had done it all. The commanding officer, chief nurse and I went to the wards, and into the sigmoid room. Of course, there were no drawers open. I was annoyed then. They opened the drawer and what did they find but the sigmoidoscope full of feces.

The next day, the chief nurse talked to me and said, "You know, you are very young." I was reassigned to the nursery out on the ramp. It was kind of nice, because that was the only place that was air conditioned. That was my punishment, in the chief nurse's own way. Everybody asked if you were out on dependents, what did you do? I guess that she felt that I was so young that I couldn't handle the corpsmen.

I really think things happened for the best. I subsequently went to the delivery room and became the charge nurse. It gave me a lasting love for maternal/child health, which I don't think I would have even thought about. As my career went on, I developed a lot of good leadership skills. I think the reassignment was the chief nurse's way of handling a problem in a way that was not traumatic to her or me. I liked it when I went to the nursery because it was a smaller cohesive group of corps personnel. I didn't have to discipline the patients. That was a biggie. You had the mothers and the babies. That's where I ended up for my career in Pensacola. I was there from December 1961 to September 1963.

I went right from active duty to reserves. My drill unit was the dispensary at Floyd Bennett Naval Air Station in Brooklyn, New York. I was with that reserve unit for about a year. Vietnam was just starting. I was doing private duty at Mary Immaculate Hospital in Queens. They would just call me when they needed me. You always had work. That was not a problem. I also was doing private duty at St. Catherine's Hospital.

The nun that had been in charge of my nursing school at St. Catherine's was now the director of nursing service at Mary Immaculate. She called me in and said, "You can't be hoboing in nursing like this." She offered me a head nurse position. Spontaneously, I said, "I think I am going back into the Navy." Consciously, I had never thought about that until that time.

I called about going back into the Navy. I had three choices. I requested New London, Quonset Point and St. Albans, twenty minutes away from home. I received orders to St. Albans. I reported on December 20. There was no leave for Christmas, but it wasn't so bad because I was home. To come back on active duty, I could get my whole physical exam at the dispensary at Floyd Bennett, except for a pap smear. The assistant chief nurse at St. Albans said, "That's okay. When you come on for active duty, we'll have you get it then." I reported aboard and went into the chief nurse. She found out that I didn't have a pap smear and was very upset. She said, "If you can't follow orders, how can you follow doctor's orders?" The assistant chief nurse was right there and said nothing. She never said that she gave the OK. I thought, "Well, I'm not going to say it either." The chief nurse almost took me by the hand down to the gyn-clinic to have my pap smear. At that point I would have really liked to have ripped up my papers and just thrown them. This was in December 1964. I was 23 years old.

I was put on the postpartum unit. That was great because I really enjoyed teaching. They weren't used to having a nurse on the OB unit that taught the corps people. I went from there to the nursery. They were having problems there with infections. I was in the nursery for about a year. Then, I developed some staph infections and could not continue to work in the nursery. I went to pediatrics.

In February 1966, I put in to go to the hospital ship. My first choice was the USS *Repose*. My second choice was Yokosuka, Japan. I got orders to Japan. I arrived in Yokosuka in September 1966. I got to Tachikawa Air Force Base near Tokyo. Someone picked me up to take me to my duty station. It was a three-hour ride from Tachikawa down to Yokosuka. The hospital had expanded from 110 beds to about 600 within a week and a half because of the Vietnam War. When I got there, they were still expanding. There was a big influx of nurses coming in. I was a lieutenant by then. Most of us were lieutenants. It was the second or third duty station for most of us. I was put on a surgical unit. The original census was initially about fifty patients. Then they put double-decker beds in the middle so that you had about ninety patients. You would get air-evacs. If your ward held ninety, you would get twenty more. You had to transfer twenty patients to the rehab unit or somewhere. Initially, we were covering two units, orthopedics and surgery.

When the wounded came in, the doctors would take off their dressings. Frequently, you had to give the bottle of Demerol to the doctor because you could not be in two places. The patients needed that before they took off the dressings. They were multi-dose vials of medication. Of course, it was absolutely illegal to do that. You really had no other choice. It was illegal because I should have been administering what I had charted out.

There have been so many changes in nursing practice since my early days in nursing, even as a student or civilian nurse. I don't think naval hospitals were that far behind other hospitals. I think they were all about the same. I used glass syringes and sharpened my own needles with a whetstone. I was responsible for cleaning the sterilizer with Bichloride of Mercury tablets dissolved in water. The IV solutions came in glass bottles with rubber diaphragms to maintain the vacuum in the bottle. Sterile dressing supplies came from central supply in packs. In Pensacola, they would make their own packs and then put them in the autoclaves. That is what was happening in Yokosuka. We had almost no disposables. Catheters were reused. They were autoclaved or boiled and came to the floor packaged in cellophane paper. They came in bulk to the hospital and were sterilized individually.

In the Navy, we were dispensing medicine out of multi-pill bottles. They used to have the round paper boxes that they used for medication with the patient's name and what the medications were. They had different sizes for the pills that were put in there. On nights, you also ordered the medication. You would write out a prescription form for any medications that patients needed.

There wasn't anything like CPR then, either. I remember a patient passing and there was nothing that you did. You just stayed with them. There was no resuscitation. We had patients coming back from surgery on to the units. There was no recovery room. Patients came back with their airways in place at times. Recovery rooms were a concept that was just beginning. As a student nurse, you may have been on alone with sixteen patients or more. I remember in nursing school, we had someone that they thought had polio. They brought an iron lung onto the unit. We had trays where we used to have to dish out the food, too. It is hard to say when we started using disposables.

In Yokosuka, there were some patients with horrendous wounds. There were a lot of shrapnel wounds. You had to change dressings twice a day until they got well debrided. Then they were sutured up. There was just one corpswave assigned to dressing changes. Some of those dressing changes were very painful. She would try to medicate patients. The patients would say, "Hey, nurse, I have pain," with a big smile on their face. That was a way of leaving behind what you were worrying about. When I first got to Japan, patients that were wounded wanted to go back into combat. As I stayed longer, they really didn't want to go back. That was from 1966 to 1968. I was there for the Tet Offensive. We got lots of casualties. It wasn't until years later that I found out we won the battle at Tet.

While I was in Yokosuka, a small intensive care unit was created. All patients were on monitors. When I was on night duty, a patient went into cardiac arrest. We started CPR, another fairly new concept, and the patient was resuscitated. Since he was on the monitor, we were able to see CPR at work.

One time, I was on night duty. We had two patients in what was called a quiet room. One was a young African American who had a week left in Vietnam. He went swimming, dove into a too-shallow pool and became a quadriplegic on a Stryker Frame. He had a beautiful body, really muscular. In the next bed was a young man that had a through and through gunshot wound to the frontal area of his brain. He was blind and spent most of the night looking for his gun. I just thought to myself, "He is going back to his parents like this. It is awful because he is not the person at all that left home." Just thinking of them, I think how awful that was. I thought it was awful then, but it seems worse looking back at it. I think it was just because we were young. You didn't have as many experiences to compare it with.

We had one young man that had a gunshot wound in the right side of his chest and arm. We were changing the dressing and hit an artery. Thank goodness, there was a corpsman there that was able to assist us. We were able to get him to the OR and saved his arm. I remember we had a top sergeant come in. He had a bullet in his carotid. He had the presence of mind to put his finger on his carotid. He was fine. It was amazing that, in battle, he had the presence of mind to take that action.

It was also sad to be holding hands with someone that really didn't want to go back. The doctors would always say, "We're not sending you back. We're just saying that you're fit for duty. It is up to the Marine Corps or whoever." I think that is the way the docs coped because they didn't want to be responsible for sending them back to the front.

That whole flower child thing hadn't taken off when I left in 1966. I remember being with a Japanese family and watching the news. It was the riots that were happening in Washington, D.C. I just couldn't believe this was my country. You kind of heard about Vietnam in 1966. It got popular in 1965–66. Before that, who even knew where Vietnam was. I do remember down in Pensacola, one flight instructor married to a nurse said he would never teach a foreign pilot everything he knew, because some day he was going to be in the skies against them. That was the truth because there were some Vietnamese pilots in Pensacola at the time going through flight training.

In Yokosuka, we got casualties from the USS *Repose* or from one of the field hospitals. They were two to five days post-injury. I used to hate the sound of helicopters coming in because that meant that you were getting a whole influx. They would call us from Tachikawa to let us know they were coming and tell how many we were getting. Most of them came in on the 3 to 11 shift. At first, it was not staffed well. Finally, when there were more nurses, there was one nurse per ward, which is what you needed on 3 to 11. For a long time, and even still, the sound of helicopters brings back the memories of air evacs. It doesn't make me anxious or nervous, or even a flashback. It is just always there. It doesn't leave you, particularly if it is the little kind of helicopter used for medevacs. There is a difference in sounds.

I went to the dedication of the Vietnam Women's Memorial in Washington, D.C. I never thought that I had any particular issues. I am not sure they were issues. I'll tell you, it brought back a lot of memories. I did a lot of crying about things and people I had forgotten.

I think the hard part of my military experiences is how many patients we sent back home without limbs. One young man stepped on a land mine, lost his foot, part of his leg and his hands. How does someone deal with that? But I didn't think about that then, partly because I was young. It was a protective mechanism. You knew it was terrible. You knew they would have a lot of rehabilitation. War is for the young, whether you are supportive or out there fighting. I think that you held the wounded to comfort them like a mother, a sister, a nurse, and talking to them. You were a little bit of everything. I was in Yokosuka from September '66 to August '68, when I went to school at the University of Pennsylvania to get my bachelor's degree.

While in Yokosuka, I covered the medical floor. I had an interesting leadership experience on the unit. You always had a ward master at arms (MAA). I wanted to make this HM3 the MAA. There was an E5 Marine sergeant who was 20 years old and very immature. They always told you that you should always have the senior person as the MAA, but you could make whoever you want the ward MAA. I made this HM3 the ward MAA. It didn't work out well at all. I went to the Marine liaison office. The top sergeant there told me to appoint that E5 as the MAA. He said, "He will function."

He came and made sure that E5 took a leadership role. That taught me a very important lesson. First of all, you do use your senior people until they prove they are not effective. Second, you need to demand the best of people. That Marine sergeant taught me a lot. I wasn't the one that was following up on him either. It was another Marine that was in his chain of command. Not many Marines in Marine liaison would have taken over the role the top sergeant did, which was very beneficial. I did learn more leadership skills, sometimes on my own by watching.

There were issues of discipline, especially in the orthopedic unit. Some of the patients would stay there for a long time. I remember sending some patients out on leave or liberty with casts. Some came back without them.

I came back to the States in September 1968. I went back to school because I knew you needed a bachelor's degree. I didn't think a degree would make me any better as a nurse. That was a time when there was a big controversy between the hospital schools and the baccalaureate programs. I did end up being a better nurse after my bachelors. It gave me tools that I didn't have before. I'm not sure it helped me technically. Psychologically, approaching people and looking at the whole person, it helped. You know how there's a curtain that goes up in your life. I remember one of the faculty at the University of Pennsylvania saying, "No one joins the organization to be the worst employee. If someone is not doing well, you need to explore that." That made a big, big impression.

After I finished school in December 1970, I really wanted to put use all these principles I learned. That was a big turning point in my life when I realized more education could make me a better nurse. I was in school two years. The University of Pennsylvania was one of the last universities to give 30 credits for your nursing school experience. I did three years in two years because I went to summer school at Temple University in Philadelphia both summer sessions. When I finished my degree, I got orders to Long Beach Naval Hospital in January 1971.

At Long Beach, I was put into supervision, which was not really what I wanted. I think I had a knack for head nursing. That's where my heart was. Now there were a lot of interesting things I thought I would like to do. I remember going in every two weeks to the chief nurse saying, "I didn't want to be in supervision." Finally, something happened that pediatrics got an opening. I became the head nurse there. That was wonderful. We did a whole lot. It was very satisfying. I got to use a lot of principles. One of the other supervisors said she had never seen a pediatric unit that was so receptive. It was just a warm feeling. People got involved and I was able to see people develop. That was a compliment to me. I am a good motivator now. I can deal with people when they're not performing, motivating them through example. I motivated myself and the corpsmen I worked with. Even the nursing aides were assisting mothers who had trouble feeding their babies.

Later, I applied and was accepted to a graduate nurse practitioner program at the University of Utah in December 1975. I was able to be involved in Navy-sponsored graduate work in pediatric nursing at the university. The project investigated pediatric weight control (Barkus, Brach, Starr, Pediatric Weight Control: Fun and Games, *U.S. Navy Medicine*, Vol. 63, May 1974, pp. 14–16).

I first came to Portsmouth after school in January 1976. I was in Portsmouth for four and a half years, leaving in September 1980. Duty at Annapolis followed, from October 1980 to October 1983, where I made captain. At these duty stations I practiced in some aspect of pediatrics or mother/baby. Eventually, I was given experience in more administrative duties as I practiced at Norfolk, Virginia, from November 1983 until April 1986. From May 1986 until December 1988 I was the deputy director of nursing for the naval inspector general. I had a wonderful, wonderful career. I retired from the Navy in 1989.

I think my faith impacted my career. I remember, as a nursing student, going into the chapel and asking God to help me be a good nurse. I think faith was a very sustaining thing for me. I couldn't imagine doing without it. I think, at times, I really do know what it means when it is said, "Blessed are the poor in spirit." Sometimes it is very hard. I have chosen to believe and I have made that leap of faith, but it's not always easy. I am a practicing Catholic.

Virginia R. Beeson

Virginia served during the last two years of the Vietnam War in a stateside naval hospital. Though some might say this short service had little value, this is where the United States Navy and the Navy Nurse Corps ordered her to serve. This is where she was felt to be of the most value. It was at this first duty station that Virginia cemented her nursing skills and understanding of basic nursing principles. It is where she formed organizational and leadership skills that would serve throughout the rest of her professional career. It is where she began to understand the importance of service to fellow members of the military and to her country.

I BELIEVE THAT GOD INTENDED for me to become a nurse. I've wanted to be a nurse as far back as I can remember. When I was little, my favorite book was the Golden Book titled *Nurse Nancy*. I used to put my dad's white business shirt on backwards and place a doily or a handkerchief with a red cross colored on it on my head. I took care of anyone who would let me practice my "nursing" skills on them—siblings, friends, and most often, pets. I know this is what God intended for me to do, and I have loved nearly every day of my career.

I graduated from High Point Regional High School in Sussex, New Jersey, in 1969. I applied to several nursing schools. I selected the University of Vermont (UVM) for several reasons. I wanted to go far away from home, but not so far that I couldn't get home periodically. It had an excellent nursing school and the campus was beautiful. It was expensive though, especially for "out-of-staters." Interestingly, the Navy had a good scholarship program. My dad knew about it and suggested that I look into this program. My guidance counselor informed me that, in addition to my four years in college, there would be a three year pay-back. I was 18 at the time. Four years in college and a three year pay-back seemed like an eternity to me. I said to my dad: "If I join the Navy, it will be four years in college and a three year pay-back. I won't be able to start my life until I'm 24 years old!" My wonderful dad said,

"Well, perhaps it's not for you." In addition, the Vietnam War was in full swing and the military was very unpopular. I went off to UVM in fall, 1969, and didn't think any more about it.

During my sophomore year, the Navy Scholarship Program came up again when a Navy recruiter came to the UVM campus and met with all the nursing students. She said, "Let us pay your way through college and you'll never have another financial worry." This time I thought about my dad. There were four children in my family. Three of us were in college at the same time; I in Vermont, my sister in Arizona and my brother in Pennsylvania. I knew it was a struggle for my parents, though they never complained. I thought, "I know! I'll go through the motions of joining the Navy, so dad will know that I'm empathetic to his financial worries, but I'm not really going to take this seriously." I got the application and half-heartedly filled it out. I had to write an essay on leadership—I was 20 years old, and as you can imagine, writing an essay on leadership was extremely unappealing! I actually wrote the essay during my European Civilization class.

I hated European Civ. I hated the idea of the essay, and thought I would get them both out of the way at the same time. After submitting my application, I had to go to Albany, New York, for an interview. The interview went horribly for a number of reasons, but I didn't care because I didn't want to be accepted anyway. On the way back to UVM, on a Greyhound bus, to make sure I had covered all bases, I prayed. I prayed that the Navy wouldn't accept me. In my conversation with God, I said that I wanted to become a nurse and practice in the best hospitals in the country. I wanted to practice with people who loved nursing as much as I did. I wanted to travel, see the world and have an exciting life. I didn't think that the Navy would be the place where these things would happen, so I prayed, "Please God, don't let them take me. This is not what I want to do."

I went back to UVM and put the Navy out of my mind. One Friday afternoon, at the end of my sophomore year, our nursing theory class was interrupted by a very excited professor who came bouncing through the door and said, "Excuse me for interrupting class, but I have a very exciting announcement to make! Ginny Beeson has been accepted into the United States Navy Nurse Corps!" WHAT!? I was beside myself! This was not at all what I wanted to do! Didn't God hear my prayer?! My friends politely clapped but looked at me with surprise, "You applied to the Navy?! When did you do that?" The Vietnam War was still going on, and the military was very unpopular. I had told no one that I applied. I asked my friends not to say anything to anybody about my acceptance. I'm embarrassed to admit that I was sad and mad. This was not my plan! However, my parents always taught me that when you take on a responsibility, you step up to that responsibility and do the best job you can. So, I resolved to "do my time," be the best nurse I could be, and get out as soon as my obligation was over. I finished my nursing program as an enlisted E5, was commissioned an ensign when I graduated, and headed to Newport, Rhode Island, in summer, 1973, for basic training.

My six weeks of training in Newport, Rhode Island, was further proof that this was a bad idea. I learned military protocols and traditions, rank structure, leadership responsibil-

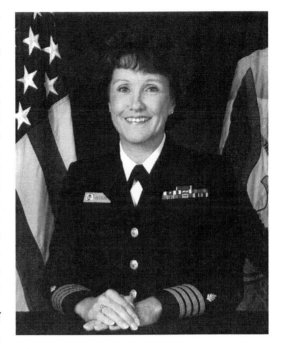

Captain Virginia Beeson served during the Vietnam era, the 9/11 crisis and Operation Desert Storm. Her example and leadership made it possible for others to perform to their potential. Photo by permission.

ities, officer-enlisted communication, marching, wearing the uniform, and the importance of physical fitness. We also learned dining etiquette, which we jokingly called "knife and fork school." I kept asking myself how marching, knowing what fork to use, and understanding the Navy rank structure would help me become a better nurse? One day they actually measured the hem of my uniform to ensure it met the three-inch standard!! Oh, right, a three-inch hem will help me become a better nurse! I hated every minute of it. Newport was beautiful and the instructors were excellent, but the drills, room inspections and marching were too much for me. One afternoon, my company officer said, "Ensign Beeson, you're taking all of this too seriously. Why don't you relax and try to have fun? Part of the drill here is seeing how you handle the pressure, adhere to routines, etc." My toleration of the routines got better, but to say it was "fun" would be a stretch.

A strong component of boot camp was leadership training and development. Instructors reinforced that we were leaders in addition to being nurses. As a matter of fact, they teach you that you are a naval officer first, and a nurse second. This did not sit well with me at all. I had wanted to be a nurse all my life. I remember saying to myself, "I will never be a naval officer first and a nurse second. I will always be a nurse first." Nevertheless, your responsibility as a leader was reinforced repeatedly in basic training and throughout my career. In every single fitness report (performance evaluation), you are evaluated on your leadership abilities. The most impressive memory I have of my initial training was the clear emphasis on leadership, that we were not only nurses, we were naval officers and leaders, and this leadership responsibility starts on day one of your career. This clear, and early, expectation of your role as nurse and leader is one of the characteristics that distinguishes military nursing from civilian nursing.

After graduating from "knife and fork school," I went to my first duty station in New London, Connecticut. It was a large submarine base that had a 100-bed hospital, the perfect size for a graduate nurse. I was assigned to a busy med-surg unit, as most new nurses were, and the opportunities for varied learning experiences were numerous. Many nurses move on from med-surg to other units, but I loved med-surg nursing. It became my specialty. I was rotated to different areas: emergency room, labor and delivery, medical unit, recovery room and the psychiatric unit. I stayed in each only long enough to discover it was not my calling. I loved that I was given the opportunity to do so many things and work in so many areas. I had countless great experiences, but I learned, in New London, that med-surg was my favorite clinical area and where I wanted to concentrate my practice.

While in Connecticut, I took a hyperbaric nursing training program for six months. Undersea medicine was a specialty on the submarine base, as there were several diver training and research programs. A common problem during diver training was decompression sickness, treated with high-flow oxygen in a hyperbaric chamber. All the nurses would be on call for divers who had health issues needing hyperbaric treatment. We had one of the only hyperbaric chambers in New England, so we also got referrals from other area hospitals. The chambers were like little submarines. We would go inside with the patient. The patient would be on a litter on one side of the chamber. The nurse would be on the other side, usually sitting on a bench monitoring the patient. The doctor would be outside the chamber monitoring everything else. The pressure and oxygen concentration in the chamber could be adjusted to help the patient recover from their decompression problems and symptoms. Completing hyperbaric training and taking care of these patients was one of many unique and challenging experiences in my Navy career.

It was in Connecticut that I really cut my teeth in nursing and became a very good clinician. I had so many different and exciting opportunities. My supervisor once said, "In the course of your Navy career, you're going to be afforded many challenging opportunities. Every time one comes your way, take advantage of it. When an opportunity comes along, be the first to raise your hand!" This was one of the best pieces of leadership advice I was ever given, and it served me well for my entire Navy career.

As stated earlier, I never planned on staying in the Navy. My plan was to do my three years pay-back and get out. I told my first supervisor again and again, "Three years and I'm out of here. This is not what I want for my professional career." However, at the end of my three years in New London, when my scholarship obligation was over, I was very conflicted. I really liked what I was doing. I was working with wonderful nurses, doctors and corpsmen; I loved meeting so many different people. I was continually amazed at how strong and collegial the nurse-doctor relationship was. I was given so many wonderful educational opportunities. I was developing strong leadership skills and enjoying the increasing responsibilities. And, I was having a ton of fun! I didn't really want to get out, but I didn't want to stay in either. In my head, my commitment to the Navy was just three years. I decided to extend in Connecticut for another year and try to decide what my next step would be.

The next year, when it was time to make a decision again, my detailer said, "You can't stay in New London anymore." My mentor said, "You can't make a decision about the Navy based on one duty station." One of my best friends said, "Gin, you can't say you joined the Navy from New Jersey and went to Connecticut!" So, I called my detailer and said, "I'd like to go to Charleston or Pensacola." I didn't know where I wanted to go, so I decided that I would let my detailer make the decision for me. She said, "Both places are open, take your pick." I chose Pensacola, and off to Florida I went! That was one of many good interactions I had with my detailer. People tell you terrible stories about detailers, but all my experiences with my detailers were great. The other title for a detailer is career planner. That's what they always were for me.

Pensacola was an interesting career change. It's a naval air station and aviators are about as different from submariners as you can get. When I went out with sub guys, they didn't talk about what they did, how important their work was, how exciting it was, or about their numerous dangerous assignments. Pilots, on the other hand, are full of stories—and bravado! They love to tell you how important their job is, how dangerous, how exciting, and how great they are at it. Although there is nothing wrong with this, it was a huge adjustment for me. I wanted to talk about how great my job was, how important, exciting and wonderful it was to be a nurse—but my story got little attention in the aviation community!

I was assigned to a med-surg unit and had my first charge nurse position, an equivalent to the nurse manager position in the civilian world. I was very good clinically and the assumption was made that I'd be a good nurse manager. As is the case in many healthcare settings, we assume that excellent clinical skills automatically translate to excellent leadership skills, but this assumption can be flawed. Leadership excellence, like all areas of excellence, comes from good training, education, mentorship and, most of all, experience. It takes time and hard work. I didn't realize this initially and felt so inadequate in the position. I felt confident making clinical decisions, assessing patients, teaching corpsmen, triaging care. Far more complex was how to deal with difficult staff members, how to manage complex communication issues, how to be courageous when unpopular decisions had to be made. I didn't like the nurse manager position at all and wanted to return to the more comfortable staff nurse role.

After six months, I went to my supervisor and said, "I don't want to do this anymore. It is too hard. Nobody likes me. I went from loving my job and everybody liking me, to hating my job and many people disliking me." I remember, one day, going by the dirty linen room and hearing one of the corpsmen talking about "Beeson, the Bitch." That's when I went to my supervisor and said, "I'm not doing this anymore. I'm not good at it. I'm not cut out for it." My supervisor was another wonderful supervisor and mentor. She said, "How long have you been in the job?" I said, "Six months, two weeks, five days, four hours and fifteen minutes, and I'm just not right for it." She said, "Obviously, I've not been spending enough time with you. I'm sorry about that. I want you to stay in the job for twelve months. I'll provide more support, mentorship and encouragement. At the end of twelve months, if you don't like it, we'll look at other options for you." Twelve months seemed like a lifetime to me, but true to her word, my supervisor was extremely supportive and did exactly what she said she would do—mentored, taught and supported me. At the twelve-month point, I didn't love the job, but I did start to feel that maybe I could do it, if I just stuck with it. I believe one of the reasons I was successful, later in my career, was having excellent mentors, teachers and supervisors in my first two duty stations. It was in Pensacola where I really started to say, "I think I do have some leadership ability. I may like this aspect of nursing. I may want to do something bigger in nursing, something beyond the clinical role." My continued and eventual passion for nursing leadership came from excellent support from outstanding supervisors.

I had another memorable experience in Pensacola. After two years as the nurse manager of the med-surg unit, I transferred to the ortho-pedic clinic. I was the manager there for a year. When I was getting ready to transfer, one of the training aircraft carriers off the coast of Florida was having medical problems and wanted a medical team flown out to them. They requested a nurse and doctor and told us their med-ical needs were orthopedic in nature. Remembering one of my earlier supervisor's words of wisdom, "Raise your hand for every opportunity!" I volunteered to go. Besides, I was the orthopedic specialty nurse! The chief of orthopedics said, "No." I was female and women weren't sta-tioned onboard ships at this time. They decided that a male nurse (with no orthopedic experience) would be the nurse on this mission. This bothered me. I appealed to my boss, and our commanding officer (CO), "You're going to send a male nurse who knows nothing about ortho-pedics, instead of me, the orthopedic nurse!? With all due respect" (a phrase you were always to use when disagreeing with someone senior), "that doesn't make sense! If we want to deliver great patient care, I should be the one to go." The answer was "no" again. This is where I practiced another of my favorite rules of leadership: "Never accept your first 'no.'" So, I said, "Could we at least get in touch with the command-ing officer of the ship and see if he would allow it. Tell him, 'The nurse that has the best orthopedic skills is a female.' Let him make the deci-sion." My commanding officer said he would make the request, but not to get my hopes up. Hallelujah! The CO of the ship said Okay! Never accept your first "No!"

The orthopedic surgeon and I flew out on a COD (carrier on-deck delivery), a tiny little plane, and landed on the aircraft carrier. It was so exciting and one of my all-time favorite Navy memories! It gave me a glimpse of the incredible dedication and service military members provide in, sometimes, very dangerous situations. The orthopod and I began seeing patients as soon as we arrived. In the mid-afternoon, after several hours of work, one of the officers asked if we'd like to watch flight operations on deck. Of course, we said "Yes"! They put us in a safe place on the back of the ship and we watched flight ops for a couple of hours. It was so exciting! Planes that land on aircraft carriers have a tail-hook, which is exactly what it sounds like—an extended hook attached to the plane's tail. The pilot's goal is to snag the tailhook on one of four arresting wires, sturdy cables woven from high-tensile steel wire, laid across the deck of the carrier to achieve a successful arrest. If they don't "catch" a hook on the first attempt, they fly off the front of the ship, come around to the back and try again. Amazingly, they don't miss very often. It was one of the most amazing and exciting experiences of my

Navy career. I watched those pilots land these huge planes on the relatively small deck of the ship. It was like nothing I had ever seen before.

When we left, we were launched off the carrier in our little plane. When you first take off, there's a dip when the plane goes down before going up. I remember thinking, "Oh my gosh, we're going into the water!" But we landed safely back at Pensacola Naval Air Station. I remember thinking how lucky I was to have had such an incredible experience. It was another reminder of all the things you get to do as a Navy nurse that you don't get to do in the civilian world. As I started to understand more about what the "real" Navy was like, it made me start thinking in a different way about patriotism, service to country and the incredible sacrifices that service men and women make in support of our nation's freedom.

I had so much fun in Pensacola, I decided that I should try one more duty station before getting out. I mean, you can't get out of the Navy without going overseas, right?! In 1980, I was transferred to Keflavik, Iceland. At the time, the primary purpose of the base in Iceland was to monitor sea and air space. There's an area in the northern Atlantic Ocean that forms a naval choke point between Iceland and the UK. On occasion, Russian subs and planes would navigate through this strait, having access to the United States border. The job of the Air Force and Navy in Keflavik was to monitor Russian submarines and aircraft that were spotted in the area, so the U.S. would be aware of their presence and activity. Whenever a Russian plane or sub entered this space, our pilots would "scramble." They would get in their planes and monitor/escort the Russian subs or planes until they were out of our air or water space. One of my farewell gifts when I left Iceland was a picture of a Russian and U.S. plane flying side by side—you can actually see the pilot's faces!

Assignment in Iceland is considered a "hardship tour" due to isolation and weather conditions. For me, it was interesting and fun! There was rigorous medical screening for all personnel going to Iceland, so most people there were healthy. I ran the outpatient clinic where we saw strains, sprains, fractures (from falls) and complaints like flu, rashes and GI issues. We did a lot of teaching on healthy life choices, stress management and preventive health. Our biggest job, on the inpatient side, was delivering babies and taking care of broken bones as a result of falls on the ice. All nurses took OR call on a regular basis for the rare appendectomy or C-section. It's at overseas duty stations that you truly learn to be a "jack of all trades."

It was in Iceland that I got a much stronger sense of the "dual role" of the Navy nurse that they talked about in basic training—naval officer and nursing professional. My responsibilities as a naval officer seemed more real and important. It wasn't nursing alone that mattered any more—there was something bigger. The military mission in Iceland was strategic and important. When the pilots got "scrambled," when their beepers went off, it meant there was Russian activity in the area. At the time, that was ominous. This started to instill in me a sense that there was a higher purpose in my work besides nursing. Our work was to take care of the sailors and airmen who did this perilous work. We had lectures about the Russian threat and our responsibility to care for our military and thereby, protect the nation. There was a Russian presence in Reykjavik, the capital. We were advised to be aware of where we went and who we talked to as we travelled around the countryside. As I learned more about our strategic defense initiatives and international relations, my sense about country, patriotism and dedication became ever stronger.

During my year in Iceland, I didn't go back to the States at all. It was just too exciting to be there. The military community was very strong. When stationed overseas, you get a true sense of being a part of the "military family." I didn't know anyone when I first arrived, and felt far away from home. Five days after my November arrival, I was at a Thanksgiving celebration where I knew no one—and everyone treated me like part of the family. Holidays were always a big deal. Everyone was invited to holiday festivities. Everyone celebrated as if they had known each other for years. When new nurses came to Iceland, they arrived at 5:30 on the "rotator," the plane that took people back and forth to the States. Every time a new nurse arrived, all the nurses, except those on duty, would go to the airport to meet her/him. If you didn't see one of your colleagues for a few days, someone would go and make sure they were ok.

On Thursday nights, the base sponsored a bus that took all who were interested to Reykjavik to hear the fantastic Icelandic Symphony— I loved that! The music teacher from the school on base would always go. On the way into the city, he would tell us all about the pieces to be played and the composers. I also loved dancing at the "O" Club on Friday nights, viewing the spectacular Northern Lights, touring the rugged beauty of the countryside with my friends, and meeting and experiencing the warmth and hospitality of the Icelandic people. While there, I was promoted to lieutenant commander, a jump from junior officer to senior officer. Shortly after putting on my "extra stripe," I got a telegram from my first supervisor in New London, now a captain, that said, "Three years and I'm out of here. Congratulations Lieutenant Commander Beeson."

The transition from nurse, to nurse and naval officer, happened subtly but certainly solidified while I was in Iceland. Although introduced to the multiple responsibilities of being a naval officer in basic training in Newport, I felt these responsibilities more keenly as my career advanced. Always aware of my responsibilities as professional nurse, I became more aware of military responsibilities, strategies, discipline, customs and traditions. I understood that I was always to be a role model for junior personnel, a representative of the United States in all endeavors, and a strong supporter of patriotic ideals. There was also a requirement to be "war-time" ready. Yearly, nurse corps officers attended a week or two of "operational readiness" training, usually at a camp in the woods. You would set up a field hospital and conduct casualty drills and operations. These expectations and activities slowly changed my feelings about my values and contributions, not just about nursing, but about my country. This dual role as professional nurse and military officer makes the role of the Navy nurse different from the role of the nurse in the civilian world. This growing sense of pride, patriotism and leadership felt good to me. I felt like a part of something much bigger than nursing.

There are other characteristics that differentiate Navy nursing from civilian nursing. One of the primary responsibilities of the Navy nurse is to train hospital corpsmen, the Navy's equivalent of the nursing assistant or primary care technician. Most units or squads that deploy in the defense of our country go with a corpsman as their primary medical care provider. These corpsmen are trained to give meds, stop bleeding, splint fractures, treat shipboard injuries, assess and treat battlefield wounds. They learn these skills from Navy nurses and physicians. Most corpsmen are 18 years old when they join the Navy. After 16 to 18 weeks of Hospital Corps School, they are assigned to a Navy hospital. Getting these young men and women ready to go out and serve in critical operational roles is one of the Navy nurse's most important responsibilities.

Another important requirement in Navy nursing is the expectation that you will move every three to four years and be ready to deploy at a moment's notice to anywhere you are needed (hospital ship, battalion aid station, foreign shore, etc.). Moving wherever and whenever almost always involves taking on more responsibility as part of the job. You could be asked to go anywhere, at any time, under any circumstance, and your answer is always: "Yes sir, or Yes ma'am, I am ready!" In the Navy, you are more than a nurse. You are a military officer serving your country. You will do whatever is asked. It was in Iceland that all these career obligations came together for me in a very meaningful way.

At the end 1981, when my tour in Iceland was over, I told myself it was time to get out. I was very proud of my Navy time and had a much clearer understanding of my roles and responsibilities, but I had never planned on making the Navy a career. My plan was always to get out. However, it's very hard to search for a job from a remote overseas duty station. What I would have to do is go back to another duty station and begin my job search from there. I was transferred to Charleston, South Carolina, where I planned to stay for a year, the maximum time you needed to stay at a new duty station before putting in papers to get out.

In Charleston, I was assigned as the nurse manager on a busy, male, orthopedic/med-surg unit. Like New London, Charleston was a submarine base. Like New London, the hospital had about 150 beds. I was a lieutenant commander now. It was clear that more leadership responsibilities were being assigned. Shortly after arriving, I was given my first real supervisory experience. After the regular day-time hours, all nursing activities were monitored by a nursing supervisor who covered the entire hospital. This was a 24-hour responsibility called the NOD, nursing officer of the day. While in the elevator one day with my NOD name badge on, a person in the elevator congratulated me on being nominated the "nurse of the day!" However, this wasn't a popularity position, it was a responsibility position and involved responding to emergencies, covering staff shortages, helping junior nurses solve problems, assisting with family challenges. I loved it! Nursing leadership resonated with me in a powerful way. Charleston provided a fabulous learning and growing experience.

After being there for a year and a half, I followed through on what had always been my original plan and started job hunting for my civilian job. I was finally going to follow through with my plan and leave the Navy. Most of my college friends had settled in Boston, so that's where I went looking for a job. I interviewed at Boston University Medical Center, Tufts New England Medical Center, Mass General, and Beth Israel Hospital. After my interview with the recruiter at Mass General, she looked at me and said, "Ginny, what are you doing here?" Confused, I answered: "I'm looking for a job." She said, "During this entire interview, the only time I've seen any excitement in your face is when you tell me about the military. When you talk about the Navy, your face lights up, your countenance changes, and everything about you is transformed. It seems to me that you love the Navy. Why are you planning on leaving it?" I thought to myself, "Oh, my gosh, I do love the Navy!" She said, "You don't want to get out, Ginny. It's so obvious that you love it."

How interesting it is that it was a civilian nurse who was largely responsible for me deciding to stay in the Navy! She was able to see in me something I felt but had never acknowledged. In my head, my plan was always to get out. I had always said that a military career was not what I wanted. All along, I was falling more and more in love with Navy nursing! I thanked her profusely, left Boston and went back to Charleston to rethink my entire career. Now it was clear that military nursing was what I loved and wanted.

At this point in my career, I was at the 10 year mark, the "do or die point" in the military, the point when you decide whether you stay in or get out of the service. Realizing how much I loved the Navy, I knew that if I was going to stay, I needed to get serious about my career. I was also starting to feel a real yearning for leadership at a higher level, for the chance to really make a difference in nursing. I decided that my next step needed to be advanced education—a master's degree.

One of the best things about Charleston was that I was no longer conflicted about what I wanted. The "stay in or get out" battle was over. I think what happened to me happens to a lot of people. You don't start out loving the Navy. It grows on you. As you do your job, meet more and more wonderful people, start to realize what all these young men and women do in support of our country and our freedom, it's no longer a job. It becomes part of you. You become part of it. You realize that, over time, you've grown into this different person. All the angst I had in Newport about being a nurse first and officer second—none of that mattered anymore. I couldn't imagine being a nurse anywhere else but in the Navy. I couldn't imagine being a naval officer and doing anything other than nursing. It no longer mattered to me which one came first. I was just one thing—I was a Navy nurse and I loved it.

I knew the next step was a master's degree. As I thought about what I wanted to pursue, nursing leadership was at the top of the list. I wanted to be a chief nurse and be able to affect change and transform aspects of nursing practice. Nursing practice in the Navy was great, but I felt it could be better. I dreamed of having my own nursing service. I applied to the Nursing Administration Program at Boston University (BU) and in 1985, when my tour in Charleston was over, I headed to Boston for the next exciting chapter of my Navy career.

Full time assignment to school on the Navy's dollar is another one of Navy nursing's greatest perks! Going to school is your full-time job—no duty, no uniform, no drills, no operational training—just study and learn—on full pay! What a golden opportunity! I hit the jackpot again when I was assigned the best advisor on the planet. She was a short, feisty, brilliant professor, mentor and motivator. After we graduated, several of us who benefited from her teaching and wisdom, said we could often hear her sitting on our shoulder, giving us advice and encouragement, firing us up to stand up for the right thing in challenging situations, and telling us to be courageous in hard situations.

My program was a two-year program including summer sessions. Navy nurses in similar situations usually went to nearby hospitals to work for the summer months. However, I had spent a lot of time in hospitals. I was going back to a hospital. I decided that I'd like to keep going to school—and Harvard had a summer leadership program! I asked my Navy school advisor if I could apply for this program. She said, "No!" I had been told "no" before, so I was not dismayed. I went to Harvard, talked to a professor, got a curriculum program, planned my classes and sent my advisor a letter. I told her how these classes would make me a better nurse and leader. I explained that while I was in Boston, I should take advantage of all the wonderful educational opportunities that Boston afforded. I said that the very best use of my summer would be more education and not going to work for two months in another hospital. There would be plenty of time for that when I graduated. She finally acquiesced. I headed to Harvard for the summer semester! Like I said, *"Never accept your first no!"*

The only downside of going to school on the Navy is that when you finish, you lose all bargaining power with the detailer regarding where you want to go. When they pay your way, and give you all that time for advanced education, you are at their mercy. So, when I talked to my detailer, I said, "I'm not picky at all. I'll go anywhere you need me. I just don't want to go to Bethesda. Please send me anywhere else." I had spent the first 10 years of my Navy career trying to avoid Bethesda. At the time, Bethesda had a reputation for being a hard place to work. It's a big hospital, extremely political, very close to Navy medicine headquarters so "Father Navy" is always looking over your shoulder, and there are "challenging" patients there. However, as I said above, I had no bargaining power. I was assigned to National Naval Medical Center, Bethesda, Maryland.

I reported to Bethesda in summer, 1987. After a terrific school opportunity, I went to Bethesda with tons of excitement and enthusiasm about putting all that I learned into practice. I was assigned as the nurse manager of a 44-bed multi-specialty surgical unit: medicine, surgery, neurology, urology and ophthalmology. It was wild and chaotically busy. Five specialties meant five sets of attending physicians, five sets of residents and multiple interns. We were always full. There was also a nursing shortage at the time. We didn't have enough staff. It was a very, very challenging assignment.

It was here that I ran into my first bad experience and the most difficult job I ever had. It was here that I fully realized the importance of really good leadership. I felt that conditions were unsafe. We had nowhere near enough nurses for the 44 patients we had. I felt that there were significant patient and staff safety issues. I didn't feel like the quality of care was what it should be. I was terribly worried about the health of my staff. I watched them work themselves to the bone. It was hard to spend time teaching and supporting the corpsmen. New nurses weren't sure they wanted to stay in the Navy after this experience.

Remembering the advice from my wonderful mentor from BU, I spoke up about things I felt were wrong, unsafe and unfair. I went to the chief nurse's office repeatedly, trying to verbalize the most important issues and offering ideas for resolution. However, I was not effective in my communication. My relationship with nursing leadership became tense and unpleasant. For the first time in my Navy career, I was miserable. I began to think that my decision to stay in the Navy was a bad one. My fitness reports were horrible—I mean horrible. When I left Charleston for graduate school, I was ranked as #1 of eight lieutenant commanders. During my time at Bethesda, I was ranked #19 of 19 lieutenant commanders.

This was the first time in my career that I hated everything about going to work. I talked to my mentor about it. She asked, "Why don't you look into leaving?" I told her that my assignment was for three years and I was stuck. She, another great mentor, said; "You are only stuck if you think you are. Why don't you call your detailer?" It's extremely unusual for your detailer to break your tour. I started thinking about it and decided to call my detailer and tell her that I'd do anything, go anywhere, to get out of Bethesda—Guam, Diego Garcia, onboard ship— anywhere. I called her and said: "When you get a job that nobody else will take, call me."

A year later (1988) she did call and said, "Do you want to be a detailer?" I said, "I don't have any idea what a detailer does, but the answer is yes!" She asked if I wanted to know what the job entailed and I said, "No, if it will get me out of here, I'll take it!" I did tell her that my fitness reports were awful. I worried that would keep me from getting the job. She said, "Come down for an interview." I went for the interview, wondering if this was a good idea. I knew nothing about detailing and had no interest in it. I just wanted to get out of Bethesda. However, I was offered the job, accepted, and left Bethesda, saying, "Goodbye, good luck. I will never, ever come back here."

The detailing job was another key turning point in my career. Being a detailer was very hard and nothing like I had ever done before. I learned so much, and again, felt the overwhelming pride of being a naval officer. A detailer is like a career counselor for Navy nurses. You try to help nurses make good career choices regarding next moves and jobs, balancing the needs of the officer with the needs of the Navy, sometimes very hard. Making everyone happy was nearly impossible, something that helped prepare me for later leadership roles. During this time, my attitude about Navy nursing, and my fitness reports, improved dramatically. I later told people that I am living proof you can get horrible evaluations and still have a great career.

One of the perks of being a detailer is that at the end of your tour, you can (usually) choose your next duty station. As I thought of my next assignment, I considered London, San Diego, Hawaii. The idea of going wherever I wanted to go was very exciting! However, during my time as a detailer, I became very aware of, and vocal about, the need for excellent leadership in health care. Things were changing in nursing and health care with the advent of managed care programs, increased mental health issues, increasing patient safety concerns, and the AIDS epidemic, to name a few. I was acutely aware of (and spoke about!) the need for strong, courageous leaders who focused on quality patient care, staff support and superb change management.

One day as I was contemplating my next assignment, my boss came in and said, "You have some good ideas about current health care issues and seem to have a passion for leadership—you need to go teach in Navy medicine's leadership program." I said, "On no, I've been thinking about my next duty station, and I've decided to go to London!" He said, "No, you're going to teach." I had no experience in teaching or education. In 1989, I set off for my next exciting career opportunity as an instructor in Navy medicine's leadership program.

After completing six weeks of facilitator training at Norfolk, Virginia, and being promoted to commander, I reported to the Naval School of Health Sciences to teach leadership principles to senior officers in the Navy Medical Department. The classes were two weeks long. I taught with a fellow medical service corps officer. The classes were held multiple times per year at various locations around the country and world. In this job, I truly got to "join the Navy and see the world!" I also learned so much more about the dedication and commitment of Navy medical department officers. They came to our classes truly dedicated to improving their leadership skills and using these skills to become the best leaders possible, thereby making Navy medicine better, stronger and safer for all who came to us for care. I often think about this now: how did they find the time to spend two weeks away from their jobs, and to stay focused? Such was the commitment to leadership in Navy medicine.

In 1995, I was transferred to Jacksonville Naval Hospital (Jax) as the assistant chief nurse for a year, and then, chief nurse. It was my first job as a chief nurse, both exciting and scary. It was the culmination of a life-time dream. I felt that this role provided the best opportunity to try and change nursing practice and really move the dial in nursing leadership. I wanted to see if I could build the kind of nursing environment I had always dreamed of. Could we build an environment where quality patient care and safety were paramount and the patient was always the center of our practice? Could I practice all the things I had learned in my graduate program and taught in the Navy's leadership program? What a rude awakening it was to learn that teaching leadership in a classroom is very different from practicing it in the real world!

Real world leadership is hard. I was overwhelmed by the multiple challenges I faced. There were so many things that I wasn't prepared for, had no experience with, and for which I had no training. For example, during my time at Jax, one of the civilian nurses committed suicide, a horrible tragedy that was hugely traumatic for all the staff. We never covered that in our leadership training. Another enormous challenge was the advent of managed care. Large health care companies like Humana and HCA were coming into the military facilities and telling us how enrolling our beneficiaries in their program would result in better care and quality of life. Managed care was a new concept that was taking hold in the civilian world. We were trying to make decisions about whether it was right for Navy medicine. Health care was changing rapidly, making challenging leadership decisions that would affect many people.

As it turned out, the Navy created their own managed care program, called TRICARE. There were several "bumps" in the rollout of this new program. The first launch of the TRICARE program excluded everyone over 65, a huge and horrible blow to people who had been promised healthcare for life when they came in the Navy. As we implemented this new program, our boss wanted members of the leadership team to go out and explain the TRICARE program to all Navy beneficiaries in the Jacksonville area. At the time, I lived at the beach and said, "I'll go to the people in my community." What was I thinking?! Most of the people in the beach community were over 65, the very people who were going to be excluded from the new managed care program.

I went to Fleet Landing, a beautiful retirement center in Mayport, Florida. The auditorium that evening was filled with seniors who were hurt, worried, anxious and very, very angry. It was a horrible evening. They were all devastated by the fact they were not going to be able to use Navy medicine for their healthcare anymore, after years in the military healthcare system. I remember thinking after that night, "I will never do that again." I could see there was something very flawed about the first generation of our managed care program. You can't renege on promises made long ago, especially to World War II, Korea and Vietnam veterans. You can't tell them, after years in a system that they have come to love and rely on, that they are being "kicked out," their term for it. I was, once again, reminded of, and in awe of, the dedication, service and sacrifice of hundreds of men and women who had given their lives and livelihood for our country. Thank Heaven the TRICARE program evolved and included the over-65 veterans. One of the biggest lessons learned while in Jacksonville was that keeping promises to those that have sacrificed life and limb for their country is very, very important.

The other challenges of the chief nurse were the usual responsibilities of ensuring quality care, patient safety, good staff morale, collaborative teamwork, sound financial decision making, career counseling, and all the other "nuts and bolts" of running a busy hospital. I was constantly reminded that being a good leader is hard, a lot harder than we make it sound in the classroom. You want to do the right thing and make everyone happy, but sometimes those two things are mutually exclusive. Often the best decisions are going to make some people unhappy. Most people in leadership (me included!) want everything to go smoothly and for everybody to be happy, but that's very hard. As a matter of fact, if everyone is happy, and everybody loves you, there's a good chance you're doing something wrong. In leadership, there will always be people who are unhappy. You need to learn to deal with that. My first chief nurse position taught me so much about people, leadership, and that translating classroom leadership instruction into the real world of leadership is very, very challenging.

In 1997, the nurse corps selected a new director. She and I were colleagues but did not know each other well. She was a "West Coast sailor." I was an "East Coast sailor." One day while in Jax, I got a call from her asking me to come and be the deputy director of the Navy Nurse Corps in Washington, under her leadership as director. In the Navy Medical Department, directors of the four medical corps are "double hatted"—i.e., they get two jobs. To help with this challenge, they have a deputy for each job. The director's two jobs were to be the inspector general for Navy Medicine and the director of the Navy Nurse Corps. I was to be her deputy for her nurse corps job. This seemed like a great opportunity for me. I returned to Washington and reported to the Bureau of Navy Medicine and Surgery in 1998.

The director of the Nurse Corps and her team develop policy and programs for Navy nurses worldwide and are responsible for all matters related to Navy nursing. For this team, the director recruited the best team of Navy nurses I have ever worked with. It was one of my favorite jobs in my Navy career. I worked with great people at Navy medicine headquarters, once again travelled around the world, helped shape Navy nursing policy and force structure, became an accomplished public speaker, met hundreds of dedicated and brilliant nurses, counselled career nurses, talked to (recruited!) new nurses entering the field, helped solve problems in Navy nursing and Navy medicine, and had many new, exciting and challenging experiences.

One of the biggest issues we faced was the debate between the certified registered nurse anesthetists (CRNAs) and the anesthesiologists on the issue of independent practice on the part of the CRNAs. As was the case in the civilian world, Navy anesthesiologists were supplemented and strengthened with excellent nurse practitioners. However, the issue of where and how they practiced became hugely contentious. Physicians insisted that CRNAs must have physician supervision, not a problem when working in land-based facilities. Anesthesia providers were also needed on ships, especially aircraft carriers. These involved 6-month deployments, assignments usually given to the nurse anesthetists, and there was no supervision when the ships were out to sea. Physicians said that was ok, no supervision was needed! Hence the challenge: how could they be independent practitioners when assigned on an aircraft carrier, but need supervision if they worked in a hospital? This was a hot topic and the subject of heated debate in the Navy medical community and the civilian world. It continues to be a topic of discussion today, as we try to understand how nurses and doctors can work together more collegially and collaboratively to meet the multiple demands of patients and the healthcare regulating agencies. The role of the advanced practice nurse has a real and very important place in healthcare. We must figure out how to maximize their talents and use them appropriately to ensure the best quality care for all patients. This was the biggest challenge I dealt with in my job as deputy director from 1998 to 2000, one that continues to be a challenge today.

My assignment as the deputy director was going to be my last tour in the Navy. The director told me that after years of doing what the Navy wanted me to do, I should choose my last assignment and go anywhere I wanted to go! So once again, I was planning my next duty station: London, San Diego or Hawaii, with a heavy focus (again!) on London. However, at the same time, the director was transferred from her job as inspector general to become the first nurse corps officer to ever be the commanding officer of the National Naval Medical Center in Bethesda, Maryland. There had never been a nurse assigned to any of Navy medicine's large medical centers, let alone Bethesda, the flagship of Navy medicine. This was an enormous and exciting challenge for her, and for the Navy Nurse Corps. She faced many challenges, leadership challenges that face the CO of any large hospital.

One day, shortly after she took command at Bethesda, she showed up in my office on the Navy medicine compound, closed the door and said, "We need to talk." I said, "No! No! Please no!" I suspected that she was going to ask me to return to Bethesda as the chief nurse. I did *not* want to go back there. I had promised myself that I would never go back. However, the admiral said those three words that nurses most often respond to, "I need you." She asked me to please think about it.

Nothing in me wanted to return to Bethesda for my last assignment. I had a thousand reasons in my head for why I shouldn't go. But at the time, my minister was preaching about hearing your "call"—what you are being called to do. Nurses at Bethesda were asking me to please come. My advisor's voice from my graduate program kept reminding me not to avoid bold challenges. Try as I might to think of all the reasons I should not have to go back to Bethesda, I kept hearing these messages that this was exactly what I was supposed to do. So, in 2000, I reported to the National Naval Medical Center, where I said I would never go again, for my last tour in the Navy.

One clear benefit of returning to Bethesda was the opportunity to work with the admiral again. She was the best boss I had ever had. I knew that working with her would be rewarding. During the entire period I worked with and for her, both at the Bureau of Medicine and Surgery and at Bethesda, she was so professional and remained constantly focused on doing the right thing, no matter what. She made all decisions based on what was right for patients first, and then for her staff, trying to understand and address the concerns that physicians had about her leadership. She was extremely team oriented and focused on making Bethesda a stronger and better place. Despite the challenges and problems posed for her, she never lost her temper or fired back at any attackers. She never succumbed to the pressure that some people exerted in an effort to make her leave. There were times when I wanted her to "fight back," appropriately and professionally, but to stand up to some of the unfair criticism. She never did. She said, "No, Ginny, we are just going to keep focusing on doing the right thing," which is exactly what she did. Eventually she won over those who opposed her and her leadership, and became one of the best commanding officers Bethesda has ever had.

I was at Bethesda for 9/11, another life-changing experience. Shortly after the second tower went down, we heard that we would be deploying the hospital ship, USNS *Comfort*, to float off the tip of Manhattan and help take care of casualties. We got the word that afternoon, and late that evening we sent 16 busloads of medical personnel to New York City to meet the ship, which had left Baltimore earlier in the day. Seeing the buses off was gut-wrenching. While we were waiting for all the necessary work to be done before they departed, all the leaders from the hospital were standing outside the buses. Suddenly, our current commanding officer (no longer the admiral) asked each one of us to get on a bus and give some words of encouragement to the troops. Although we had no idea what we were going to say, we each hopped on a bus. After such an awful day, I stood on the bus for a few moments trying to gather my thoughts. I then offered a few words of encouragement, support and confidence, and asked if anyone had any questions. Someone asked, "Captain Beeson, how long will we be gone?" I had to reply that I wasn't sure. The second person asked, "Captain Beeson, what will we see in terms of injuries?" And once again, I had to say that I wasn't sure, but most likely burns, inhalation injuries, shock, etc.

The third question was, "Captain Beeson, do you think we are prepared to take care of these casualties?" This question was easy for me. I told them that I had complete and utter confidence in them. I reminded them that we had all had years of training for combat care, and this would be similar. I reminded them of how smart, dedicated and experienced they were. I told them they would get whatever support and help they needed from us. We would be talking to them regularly, and praying for them daily. There was a lull in the communication and complete silence on the bus. I was so distraught that I didn't seem to be able to give them the answers and assurance I knew they wanted. How long they would be there, when they could come home, what would they face, etc. However, in the lull of the conversation, someone from the back of the bus shouted, "Don't worry, Captain Beeson. We are ready!" to which the entire bus responded "Yes, we are ready."

It made me cry that day on that bus; it makes me cry today. The dedication, unwavering commitment and complete willingness to do whatever is asked of them, to go wherever they are asked to go and do whatever they need to do, on a moment's notice—and having no idea what they will face, or when they will return, is a hallmark of people in the Navy Medical Department and makes me burst with pride that I am associated with these kinds of heroes. It demonstrates patriotism and service to country beyond anything I have ever known, and that day, on that bus, will forever be one of my best memories of my Navy career.

Another challenge during the 9/11 crisis was staffing the hospital after most of my staff left on those buses. Fortunately, news that the USNS *Comfort* was deploying got out quickly. When it did, nurses from all over the city called and offered to help. First and foremost, were the wonderful civilian nurses who were on staff at Bethesda. Every one of them responded, coming in, calling in, and telling me that they would do whatever was needed to keep things running smoothly—and they did, working many long hours. The civilian staff who work at military hospitals are the "glue" that holds everything together when active-duty troops deploy. They are also heroes in my book.

Also, quick to respond were other area military nurses. The chief nurses from Walter Reed Army Medical Center, and Malcolm Grow Air Force Medical Center both called and asked what we needed, saying, "We'll send you anything you need and we'll send it right away"—and they did. The National Institutes of Health (NIH) is right across the street from Bethesda and the chief nurse there called and offered help. Retired nurses from all over the area called in, many saying, "I can't work clinically anymore, but I can be a runner, assist patients, pass trays, answer call lights." Nurses in school called and offered to help. Civilian hospitals around the city offered help and staff. The response was overwhelming in terms of the number of people who responded with help and support. It was a dramatic example of everyone pulling together in a time of crisis. The Pizza Hut down the road delivered 50 pizzas!

My most memorable call was from a lieutenant commander from San Diego who was in Washington on vacation. She called and said, "Captain Beeson, I'm here in DC on vacation from San Diego. I've called my chief nurse who said to report immediately to you, do whatever you need me to do, and stay for as long as you need me to stay. What do you need me to do?" I said, "Well, what is your job in San Diego?" She said, "I'm the nurse manager in the intensive care unit." This was an answer to prayer for me because nearly every one of my ICU nurses had left to staff the USNS *Comfort*. I asked her, "Can you come and run my intensive care unit? I have Army, Air Force and NIH nurses up there who have never been in a Navy hospital." She said, "Don't you worry Captain Beeson, I AM THERE!" I hung up the phone, said a quick prayer of thanks, and got back to work. About five minutes later the phone rang again, and it was the same nurse. She said, "Captain Beeson, I have no idea where you are!" This is another great example of the dedication and sacrifice of dedicated military professionals. They are willing to go "there" when they don't even know where "there" is. Such is the dedication of Navy nurses.

The Iraq War also started while I was at Bethesda. Once again, we deployed many of our nurses and corpsmen to duty stations in the Gulf in support of this effort. The reserves came in to "backfill" and augment our staff. My last year and a half at Bethesda were spent managing a mix of active duty and reserve nurses. Luckily for me, a senior Reserve Navy Nurse Corps captain was also assigned to Bethesda to help me manage this large and varied staff. To my great delight and surprise, the reserve nurse assigned to help was a classmate of mine from my college days and the person I had joined the Navy with on the Buddy Program in 1971! Although she got out after two duty stations and joined the reserves, we continued to be best friends for our entire careers. She and I worked together and ran the nursing department at Bethesda during this very stressful time. Being stationed with her again was another wonderful benefit of my Bethesda experience. I started my career with her, and I ended my Navy career with her—how cool is that?

A very short time after the war started, we began getting troops back from the war, injured and in need of care. They were usually flown to Andrews Air Force Base in the late evening and arrived at our hospital around midnight. When they first started arriving, our commanding officer wanted one of the board members to be present to ensure everything went smoothly for these wounded warriors. The most seriously injured would arrive in our emergency department. Those less seriously injured, the "walking wounded," would arrive on a bus, configured to be an ambulance, holding about sixteen patients. One evening when I had duty, the bus arrived at the front of the hospital and the men got out and headed for the front door. One of them, however, started walking away from the bus and away from the hospital. The security guard called him back saying, "Marine, come back. This is the entrance." The young Marine waved him off saying, "There is something I need to do." The security guard was agitated and told me to order him back to the entrance of the hospital. The Marine had a walking cast on his leg and an airplane cast on his arm. I knew he wasn't going to be able to go far. I told the security guard to let him go. The young man walked over to the grassy lawn, knelt down and kissed the ground. It brought tears to my eyes and the eyes of everyone who saw it, including the security guard. The Marine then came over to me, stood at attention with his casted leg and arm and said, "Thank you, Ma'am." It's another thing I will never forget.

We had a lot of challenges while I was at Bethesda: a fire at Walter Reed Army Medical Center brought dozens of patients to our facility; 9/11 and trying to staff the hospital after hundreds of our staff left; caring for the returning casualties; instituting a service line organizational structure; meeting quality, safety and service metrics; managing the needs of multiple congressmen, generals and admirals, and most importantly, handling the needs of all the enlisted men and women, who every day work so hard for our country and all that we hold dear.

Although I never wanted to go back to Bethesda, it turned out to be the perfect way to end my Navy career. To have the chance to be back in the hospital, which I love, and to work with the best and most dedicated nurses in the world, doing the most important job in the world—caring for soldiers, sailors, airmen and Marines who put their lives on the line every day, so that we can enjoy all of our freedoms, was the best and most fitting end to my Navy career, one that was filled with great privileges, opportunities and adventures.

I retired from the Navy in June 2003. In my retirement remarks I told the audience about my prayer long ago on that Greyhound bus, when I prayed that the Navy wouldn't accept me. I know that God heard my prayer on that bus in 1971 because, as is often the case with prayer, I didn't get anything I asked for, and everything I prayed for. I wanted to practice with the best nurses and doctors in the world, in the finest hospitals in the world, and to travel and meet the most dedicated people in the world—and God dropped me in the lap of the Navy medicine family, who cared for me beyond all expectations, for 30 wonderful years.

Go Navy!

Carol Keith Brautigam

Carol found that her naval experience expanded her world view and that strong teamwork supported her through difficult times.

BORN IN 1944, I GRADUATED from high school in Charles City, Iowa, in 1962. I knew I wanted to be a nurse. There weren't many women in health care at that time. It was the era where you were either a nurse, secretary, or teacher. In 1962, there were few baccalaureate programs in the country not associated with a university. My original thought was to go to a university program. I was encouraged by my high school English teacher to look for a smaller college. Most of the four-year programs were three-year, hospital-based, diploma programs. Then, you attend two more years at a college to earn your baccalaureate degree. There was a college in southern Minnesota, St. Olaf College in Northfield, with a stellar nursing program. I chose this program because it incorporated nursing in all four years of college.

The Vietnam conflict was going on. Nurses were in demand. The military offered to pay for two years of your college for three years of service after you graduated. When the military nurse recruiters came to St. Olaf College, I didn't attend the meeting. I was not very interested. But my roommate was really interested in the Navy. She came back from the meeting all excited and encouraged me to go with her for an interview with the recruiter in Minneapolis. After the interview I was "sold" on nursing in the U.S. Navy Nurse Corps.

Upon graduation from St. Olaf, I went to Officer Candidate School in Rhode Island for six weeks. My first duty station was Chelsea Naval Hospital, Massachusetts. The original hospital was built before the Civil War. A three-story stone building with thick, thick walls served as the female officer quarters on the campus. The hospital itself dated from pre–World War II and was a three-story brick building. Sadly, the entire campus is no longer there.

I was part of a twelve-ensign nurse group stationed at Chelsea. We were required, as new young officers, to live on base. The living quarters in that original hospital had community kitchens at either end of the building. Those on the third floor had skylights because they had been the original operating rooms where surgery was done by daylight during the Civil War. There was a basement and a subbasement. In the subbasement were cells. That was a great place for Halloween ghost stories. We wondered, "Was this where they kept the insane chained?" or "Was this part of the underground railroad?"

Soon, there were more and more nurses arriving at Chelsea Naval Hospital. Not all could be housed on campus. A note posted in the staffing room read, "Nurses are needed to live out." A new friend was from Rockport, Massachusetts, and knew Boston well. With her knowledge, we located to an apartment in Beacon Hill, Boston, just off Charles Street. As we were the first to move off campus, there was a big discussion among the nursing staff about whether we could wear our bridge coats over our nursing whites while on public transportation. We took the MTA and then a bus, which let us off at the hospital gate. There was a three-block walk from the gate, uphill to the hospital, which overlooked the Charles River. Boy, was that ever a windy walk, especially the wind coming off that river in winter! We did wear our bridge coats and all other paraphernalia when we were on the public transit. We loved being in Boston. Living "off base" gave us a sense of freedom that was a little different than when we lived on base.

I was assigned to sick officers' quarters (SOQ), a medical/surgical unit on the third floor of the main hospital. I cared for an admiral, some Navy captains, and both young and older officers from all branches of the military. Military patients were assigned to military hospitals as close to their homes as possible. Whether it was an Army, Navy or Air Force facility was not as important as where the soldier's home was located.

Some patients arrived as soon as 96 hours after their injury. If there were major fractures, such as a femur injury, they had been transported from Clark Air Force Base, Philippines, to Travis Air Force Base, and then to all points in the States.

At this time, military hospitals still had open wards of 20 to 30 patients each for enlisted personnel. Officers on SOQ had private rooms. The nurses' station was a room all by itself, not a cubicle in the middle of the ward. The office had a door and was simply furnished with a couple of desks and a chart rack.

Attached to the hospital were several wooden ramp wards. Constructed for the Korean War wounded, they were damp and smelled old, but were full of enlisted patients that were too many to be housed in the brick hospital. One ramp ward was only for isolation of wounds and infectious disease, such as TB. I worked on the officers' quarters for half a year. Then, I was assigned to an orthopedic unit in one of the ramp wards. A plus for those patients was that those with body casts or in traction for long weeks could have their beds rolled outside where they could get some much-needed sunshine during the warm months of the year. To put things into perspective, at the same time the naval hospital had open wards, Massachusetts General Hospital was the same. Patients were all in one big room with a bathroom at the end.

The enlisted wards had a little cubicle for the nurses' station where the charts were kept. If you were really sick, your bed was pushed right by that station. As you got better, you got further away. So, patients knew how sick they were and how well they were recovering. Because military personnel would be sent back to duty, if possible, the nurses assigned enlisted patients to jobs on the wards. We had one patient that had lost an arm. He was so depressed. We nurses had him go with us in the daytime to make beds. It truly helped his morale to contribute to others. Men in wheelchairs could make the rounds to each patient on the ward and get a list of what everybody wanted from the gedunk, which was like a little store. At the gedunk, hamburgers, chips, junk food, combs, etc., could be purchased. Recovering patients could line waste baskets with paper bags. Once patients were well enough to leave an inpatient unit, they went to an outpatient unit, where more manual work on the hospital grounds and on equipment was required. This helped them to be fit to return to full-service duty, including possible deployment to Vietnam. During the convalescent period they were no longer patients, but were assigned to the hospital until ready to go back to their unit. That determination was made by a physician.

On my annual evaluation, I checked the box asking to be assigned to a hospital ship. I received that assignment to the USS *Sanctuary* (AH-17). There were two hospital ships, the USS *Sanctuary* and the USS *Repose*. My trip to the ship began with a plane flight from Travis Air Force Base, California, to Da Nang, Viet Nam. Enroute, the plane stopped in Alaska to pick up supplies and refuel. There was a stop in Okinawa to let off military, take on military and refuel. Flying over Tokyo, one of the pilots said to look out and see the lights of the city. It was a huge glow of light. Later we landed in Da Nang. It had been about a thirty-hour plane ride.

We landed in Da Nang during the day. A Navy chief told me the USS *Sanctuary* had sailed that morning for Subic Bay, Philippines. He drove me, in a jeep, to the Da Nang Naval Hospital. There, the chief nurse said, "Well, the ship will be back in ten days. You can stay here and work until it comes back." That sounded good to me, a rather "wet behind the ears" Navy officer. At the officers' club, I saw a surgeon who had been at Chelsea and we recognized each other. He said, "What are you doing here?" I said, "Well, I missed my ship because my flight was delayed." He said, "Oh, you should get a helicopter to Phubai, take a plane to Clark, then to Subic. You should meet the ship in Subic Bay." It had just been the Tet Offensive, so I wasn't really excited to do that. Since the chief nurse said I could stay at the hospital, that's what I did.

Despite having made an inexperienced decision, it was an interesting and informative experience. Naval Hospital Da Nang had quonset huts with cement floors that could be scrubbed down. The huts were air conditioned. I had a chance to work in the ICU and see what was happening with injured coming in fresh from the field.

When the ship came in, I took a boat out to it. The little transport boats came alongside the ship where you climbed a ladder to come aboard. The ship was rocking a little bit, even though it was in the harbor. Climbing aboard was a little tricky. The chief nurse on the ship, a captain, said to me, "Where were you!?" I told her about the chief nurse's offer to stay there until the ship came in. She understood how my inexperience had allowed me to accept the offer. After a year and a half at Chelsea Naval Hospital, I was on board the USS *Sanctuary* (AH-17).

In the 1960s, the *Sanctuary* and *Repose* were renovated at $20,000,000 each. They did a lot of work to get these ships to become hospital ships. They had been transport ships in Korea and World War II. They were not hospital ships. Renovated, they carried a full ship's crew, 450 patients, plus all the hospital crew. Each ship had three operating rooms, a recovery room and an intensive care unit (ICU). There were physician specialists in internal medicine, neurosurgery, anesthesiology, general surgery, and orthopedics. Nursing specialists included certified nurse anesthetists, operating and recovery room nurses, central supply nurses, and general medical-surgical-orthopedic nurses. There were pharmacists, chaplains, liaison officers with the other branches of the services. There were American Red Cross representatives who did social service work.

The patients on the internal medicine wards were in bunks that were three high. If you were pretty sick you were in the middle. As you got better you went up to the top. When people got discharged, they went to an area in the hold of the ship where the beds were five high. People had to be in good physical condition to climb. A lot of them were going to go back and fight again. We had three areas for the sickest patients where there were single beds. That was in the orthopedic area, where they had traction, the ICU, and ten beds on the medical ward for the sickest patients, most with malaria.

In the nurses' quarters, we had a little lounge, our own bathroom and showers and our own state rooms. The state rooms were all bunk beds, except mine. The one I was in had three beds, one bunk bed and one single. I got the top bunk, appropriately since I was a LTJG and my two roommates were full lieutenants. As officers, we ate in the dining room of the ship known as the ward room. The ward room had long tables with white linen cloths and napkins and a full array of silverware for the three meals. We were served individually by the ship stewards. There were enough officers between the ship crew and the hospital crew that there were two sittings: the junior officers ate first.

For the first several months there was so much to talk about: work, when we would go to Subic Bay next, the Fourth of July, a presidential election, Thanksgiving, Christmas, where everyone was going for their R&R break. We junior officers had to be chased out of the dining room to make way for the senior officers. By the end of our year on board (January–March, when the crews turned over), we could eat a full course meal in 15 minutes. The enlisted men (and all were men) ate in a cafeteria below decks. Often times, nurses would choose to eat a meal with the "crew" to show appreciation for the work the corpsmen and ship's crew were doing.

The cooks were primarily Filipino. They were excellent. But they were not used to a hospital ship where people didn't show up on time for a meal. You had to be really astute and take the time to call down to ask them to save you a meal if you weren't going to get there. Otherwise, your meal would not be saved for you. Pretty quickly, the cooks learned that all the nurses and doctors wanted to eat, but they might not be able to get there. They might not even have time to call down. They learned to save meals for any officer not showing up in the ward room. Working nights, you could go to the kitchen/galley and the cooks would make anything you wanted. I enjoyed wonderful fried rice!

There was terrific teamwork on the ship. Most of the time physicians, nurses, corpsmen worked 12 hour shifts. In the States, at the time, it was still eight-hour shifts. On the ship, if your shift started at 7:00 a.m., you worked until 7:00 or 8:00 p.m., depending on how long report took between shifts. I was working on internal medicine which had a usual census of 120 patients. Even if all you did was to note that your most well patients were there, it took a while to give a report on that many people. Even for the sickest patients, there wasn't time for much of a report. The goal was to get off for the 8:00 p.m. movie in the ward room. These were mostly Class B westerns. A big event was seeing Paul Scofield in *A Man for All Seasons*. For the ship's crew and patients, there were movies on the upper deck at night.

The two hospital ships sailed in opposite directions. One would begin in Da Nang. One would be at the DMZ. They sailed north and south along the South China Sea coast between Da Nang and the DMZ. Both ships were painted white, with three large red crosses on the sides, and had their running lights on, meeting the Geneva Convention requirements. Even when following a task force at night, our running lights were on. The hospital ships moving along the coast allowed the hospitals to be closer to battle action and quicker trips to the hospitals with those wounded.

There were two large Navy hospitals in country, Da Nang Naval Hospital and Saigon Naval Hospital. On the ships, patients were brought by helicopter. They were loaded from the fighting area onto the helicopter by corpsmen and other personnel. Anyone brought to us was cared for. In addition to American troops, we had North and South Vietnamese, North and South Korean, Chinese, Australian, French and Canadians. We had women and children. There was an international ward dedicated to the women and children.

Many of the Vietnamese people's homes were destroyed. They lived in temporary, paper-like houses. Because they cooked with oil lamps, these houses would catch fire easily. We had several burn patients among the children and women. The Navy chief in charge of food service was a single man who just loved little kids. He would gather up all the kids that were ambulatory and take them into the ship's store. They would get popcorn and candy. Then, he would take them to the movies. The chief was often seen walking about the ship with a trail of kids following him. We had some of the children there for a long time. Six-year-olds would be the size of an American three-year-old. Their nourishment hadn't been good but they were smart and picked up English very quickly.

We all worked as many days as we needed to. You might work many days in a row. The chief nurse tried to give nurses days off. For recreation, once you were off duty, a visit to the ship's store was often on one's agenda. It wasn't like a Target, where you have aisles of items. It was a small area. Cassette tapes were just out. What you probably bought was a reel-to-reel tape recorder with speakers or you would buy the little, tiny cassette tape recorder. American Airlines tapes were copied by everyone. They were a big deal. American Airlines was the first airline that really provided music for passengers to listen to. They sold their tapes of music. Somebody on the ship would buy some American Airlines tapes. Then, everybody would copy them. You weren't supposed to be doing that, of course. But Vietnam was not a declared war at the time. It was a police action. No one cared enough to turn people in for copying tapes. Cameras were another big item because it was fun to have them, and they didn't require storage. Officers had space in their state rooms for some storage. But if you bought speakers for your tape deck, the crew found a place, probably above the pipes somewhere on the ship, to store them for you. For individual space, the crew had a bunk bed with drawers beneath. Another recreation area for officers was the officer deck on level with the wheel house at the top of the ship. Sunbathing in swim suits was a relaxing and social event.

The ship's enlisted crew was required to consistently work 12-hour shifts. Occasionally the hospital census was low enough that patient care shifts were eight hours. To match the ship's crew requirement, the hospital corpsmen worked an additional four hours in the laundry.

Everyone looked forward to the 90-day rotations to Subic Bay, Philippines, where the ship went for regular maintenance. Prior to sailing, as many stable patients as possible would be off-loaded at Da Nang, flown to Clark Air Force Base and home from there. This allowed everyone to have three days of liberty in Subic. Plans were made for day trips to Baggio in the mountains and other destinations off base.

Salt water is the enemy of steel ships. They must be repainted, inside and outside, on a regular basis. Trips to the Philippines with fewer patients allowed for the interior painting. There were two captains aboard. The captain of the ship and the captain of the hospital. The captain of the ship had priority over the hospital captain. Prior to sailing, the captain of the ship would go through the wards looking for enlisted personnel who were willing to stay aboard, to help paint the ship in exchange for liberty in Subic. All the enlisted patients who were well enough to be living in the hold of the ship, with their bunks five high, would be working in the laundry or somewhere on the ship. Those would be offered five days of liberty if they would help paint the ship going and coming from Subic Bay. Of course, they would do that, because nobody really wanted to go back to the rice paddies to fight. You always had enough patients who decided to help paint the ship. The five days of liberty in Subic Bay was exciting. The base in Subic had bowling alleys, golf courses, tennis courts, swimming pools and Olongapo Bay. It was a little town that was supported by the sailors and soldiers having liberty in Subic.

The ship had pharmacists on board and about five techs that worked with them. When it came to IV medications, we mixed our own. There were no hoods or filtered needles for glass vials. In fact, there were no angiocaths either for IVs. You started your IVs with just a regular 18 or 20 gauge metal needle. It was exciting on the ship when we got the first intercatheter. They are almost like a PICC line because they were so long. The cannula was on the inside of the needle, so when you made your puncture, the hole was bigger than the cannula. They had a long cannula so that the fluid coming out of the tip was quite a distance away from the puncture hole to try and prevent leakage. There was a green plastic piece that secured the needle and was taped onto the forearm. You'd probably use an antecubital vein for the puncture. That was the big new thing. The other big new thing they had come out with was Sulfamylon for burns. That really stings when it goes on and upsets electrolytes. It was several years before they got Silvadene cream figured out.

There was a six-year-old little boy in the ICU, but the size of a three-year-old. He had extensive burns. Each day he smeared himself with his own feces. In order to clean him off, the corpsmen would wash him off in the utility sink. They could stand him up under the faucet and have the soil wash down the drain. Afterward they reapplied the Sulfamylon, a painful, stinging process. That happened every day. One Sunday, when we were in Da Nang, a boat came out to our ship. Local Vietnamese civilians were sometimes patients on the ship. The boat would come out and families would come visit. His parents came out that day. The ICU staff quickly sent for the interpreter to find out why this boy was soiling himself every day. Well, he had never had a shower before. It was so wonderful for him to be under the warm running water that he would endure getting washed off and having the Sulfamylon reapplied. We just about all cried.

The respirators we had were the Bird Box respirators. It was a little box delivering pressure without any volume. We had a couple of circle electric beds in ICU. At the time we thought we were pretty advanced, but when we look back, we realize how creative we had to be with what we had. We had one cardiac monitor on the ship; CPR was in its infancy at that time. The hospital ships today have 1000 beds, 12 ORs and 100 monitors plus whatever is in ICU. We all learned it. Some staff had prior duty at the Naval Hospital Philadelphia, where they had been doing research about whether CPR should be done with hand compressions or whether it was more effective to use a machine.

Abdominal wounds are very difficult. They drain and drain. Many times, we would use a circle electric bed for them. We lined the bedpan hole with a plastic bag. The wound was left open/undressed and the patient turned onto his abdomen to let the wound drain into the bag. These patients were not well enough to stand up in a shower. It was hand-irrigating open wounds or draining them on the circle electric beds. You just wanted to get all that ooze out of there for a little while.

We were not able to follow many patients to see what happened to them. There were too many coming and going. Once in a while, the physicians would really try and track what happened to somebody. There was one man on the ship for months with severe abdominal wounds they were able to track. This patient almost died several times. We finally transferred him out because we just wanted to try to get him home. He did get home to see his family before he died.

The hardest day I ever had in ICU was when we had taken on land mine injuries. In land mine injuries, people lose arms, legs, eyes. There is head trauma. Often there are multiple amputations. Working with these patients was very difficult because the injuries were so extensive. In the ICU that day were all new corpsmen, straight from corps school, and only one seasoned corpsman to assist nurses. It was a traumatic first day for those corpsmen.

Malaria was a common disease in Vietnam. I watched two patients die from it. The red blood cells burst open and all that hemoglobin is released, plugging up the kidneys. They would die from kidney failure. We had one dialysis machine on the ship.

The blood and any medications or IV fluids that were outdated, just like in the States, were not used. There is really a little leeway that we couldn't take advantage of on the ship. But the U.S. State Department Hospital in Da Nang, for civilian casualties, did use the outdated supplies the hospital ships provided them.

Once in a while, we did an underway replenishment. That is how we got our fuel and supplies. They'd put the fuel lines between the ships to fill the ship with fuel. Sometimes they would send pallets of different items back and forth. Mainly we got supplies when we went into Subic Bay or Da Nang. One day, a ship come alongside and the captain came over. He didn't go to the captain of the hospital. He went to the captain of the ship. He said, "Captain, I'm going to take some of your nurses over for lunch. Who's available?" Four of the off-duty nurses went over in a chairlift on a rope slung between the ships. The captain asked the nurses, "What do you need?" One of the nurses said, "We could use a foot bath." It was hard about showers and water because the ship desalinates its own water. When malaria patients with 107-degree temperatures were put into the shower to cool down, the ship's crew would be so upset because we were using so much water. We told them there was limited time to cool these patients to avoid brain damage. The showers were the fastest way.

The supply ship was going into Subic Bay. Somebody went into Manila and saw, not a foot bath, but a real bathtub, and bought it. The tub was blue. The USS *Sanctuary* received it during an underway replenishment along with one pallet of lettuce. The chief engineer said, "Well, you girls can have this bathtub in your bathroom, but we aren't hooking it up. We cannot have water used that way." A few weeks later, we were in Subic. Someone had communicated to the supply ship what the chief engineer had said. On the wharf was a band playing and a claw footed tub being raised and lowered on a crane. It read the name of the chief engineer and "Folly." During the time in Subic, someone from base installed the tub. We filled the tub with water and bubbles. One of the more petite nurses got in wearing her swimsuit. We nurses held open house for the bathtub and allowed the crew to come through the nurse's quarters to see the bathtub. The blue bathtub was a fun event, a morale booster. It was never used for a real bath by anyone.

During our tours, everybody had five days of R&R. There were specific places you could go: Bangkok, Hawaii, Hong Kong, or you could go to different places in South East Asia. You couldn't come back to the States because that was too far. I went to Hong Kong for five days. Some of my experiences there were eye-opening: the boat people, the shacks on hillsides, that chicken was simply cubed so some pieces had bones in them, the gambling with mahjong. While I was in Hong Kong, I stayed at the Hilton and received a military discount. I walked around, took cabs and red doubledecker buses around the city and tried to keep track of where I was. I ate local food and did some shopping. I had some shoes, handbags and a suit made. Other officers had been there. They told me locations to go for different things.

On my way back to the States, I did a "delay in route" and stopped in Japan, where one of my classmates from St. Olaf College was stationed. I spent some time in Japan with her. We went to the northern part of Japan, around Kyoto, and toured there. It was March, and there were people on the bullet train going north. Many were going skiing. I hadn't realized there was skiing in Japan. We stayed in a local place where the windows were like rice paper and there wasn't any heat. We took a hotsie bath before going to bed so our bodies were all heated up. At the foot of the feather bed was a crockery piece, almost like a flower pot, but it was a cylinder inside a corduroy sack. It had been heated, and placed by our feet so we were toasty warm when we got into bed. We stayed warm all night.

We went out to a little fishing village island, walked around and saw some of the tourist attractions. The Japanese farmers had little tiny trucks in their fields. They looked like Model A trucks. They were about as long as a dining room table. In Tokyo, the traffic was just wild. Driving was on the left side, but everyone also used the right side of the road to weave in and out of whatever was blocking their way. We had some pretty wild rides.

The tour on the ship was one year, March 1968 to March 1969. My delay en route in Japan was ten days before returning to Travis Air Force Base. I finished out my Navy career at Great Lakes Naval Hospital, outside of Chicago. It is a large hospital with a corps school for training corpsmen. I was assigned to an internal medicine ward. The care was not different from what I had done at Chelsea or on the ship for internal medicine. July 1969 I was discharged from active duty in the U.S. Navy Nurse Corps from Great Lakes Naval Hospital. My three years in the U.S. Navy Nurse Corps remain a highlight in my 43-year nursing career. In addition to the memories, I became lifelong friends with some shipmates.

In reflecting on my Vietnam experience, the hospital ship immediately narrowed my focus as I stood for the first time in "my" three-bed stateroom in the Women's Officer Quarters. Ahead of me was a white sink. To the left was a set of bunk beds and across from them a single bed. To my right were two desks with storage bins and a chair each, across from them a single desk, chair and three lockers. All were metal construction, painted grey. I began to sense the slow rocking of the ship at anchor in Da Nang Harbor. Coupled with a slight diesel fuel smell I began to feel a bit queasy. I was quiet and then felt myself saying, "I can do this for a year."

"This" was being a nurse on a hospital ship that received war injured GIs and others, often within minutes of injury. Patients arrived by helicopter. Patients were my whole world, affecting how many hours I worked and what I thought and dreamed after work. While patients at Chelsea Naval Hospital might arrive as soon as 96 hours after injury, often times needing a first bath, my focus was directed both at the hospital experience and the Boston experience where I had lived on the back side of Beacon Hill. Now my world was the ship, its patients and my co-workers.

I believe my patient focus was like the other 31 nurses, physicians and corpsmen. The ship's officers and crew were focused on maintaining a well-run ship that served as the hospital. The result was an extremely strong bond among the hospital and ship personnel. We quickly became a strong, cohesive team that supported each other as we cared for patients and the ship. It was a model of people giving their ALL for one purpose, one goal. It was years before I experienced other teams that were as strongly knit. Those were during work stoppages (read union strikes) where sometimes I was on the picket line and sometimes inside as management.

But while my focus narrowed, my worldview was expanded as we cared for men (mostly), women, and children in the tight quarters of the ship. Several countries, cultures and languages were present. Some did not speak English. Pantomime and an interpreter were needed in caring for them. When a few women became well enough to get around the ship, they were allowed to cook their own food on a charcoal burner at the fan tail of the ship. Nurses (the other available women) were invited to partake of the cooking. How refreshingly prepared with new spices were the greens, chicken and pork. It was my introduction to another culture's food. That introduction has stayed with me in enjoying foods from around the world ever since.

My expanded worldview included wonderful, multiple examples that "people are people" everywhere. But, the results of armed conflict were often devastating in caring for the wounded, no matter who they were or how they had been injured. Civilians suffered as greatly as soldiers. What was accomplished with the damage to persons, housing, foliage in a country of beautiful scenery and waterfalls? A consideration of "why war," as the United States has been so involved with war over our entire history has occupied my thoughts for years. While on the ship I received a letter from a college classmate saying, "Carol, you tell what you are doing, but you don't tell what you are thinking." I angrily wrote back, "Don't you understand? If I thought about it, I couldn't do it."

It was the strong team that helped me to do it, through difficult days when land mine injuries arrived, when young men died from malaria, when we went through a typhoon. Part of the team has stayed with me through the years in ship reunions and in close friends with whom I still connect.

Gloria and John (Jack) Caffrey

This account is a combination of two accounts, those of a married Navy couple; Gloria's is in regular Roman type; Jack's is *italicized.*

I GRADUATED FROM Illiana Christian High School in Lansing, Illinois, in 1967. I decided on nursing because my high school was a college prep school. Of my possible career choices, what appealed to me was nursing. I have to credit my chemistry teacher with helping me make that decision. I was good at math and science. He thought nursing might be a good avenue for me.

Coincidentally, he convinced my best friend to go to nursing school. We were accepted at a school that unexpectedly closed their program two months before the school year was supposed to start. The teacher stepped in again to help us. Another daughter graduated from West Suburban Hospital School of Nursing in Oak Park, Illinois. He contacted the dean of the school and said, "I have two students that, unexpectedly, don't have a school." She said, "Send them up and we will interview them." Between my chemistry teacher and the dean, we had a place to go. It was a three-year diploma program.

I lived at the school with the dorm mothers and 10:00 p.m. curfews. It was all girls. It was a very good school, very high academic standards. At one point, I went through what most students go through, not being sure nursing was for me. However, I decided to stick it out. It was very difficult. I was good at math and science, but I wasn't particularly good at rote memorization. There was a lot of it, especially anatomy and physiology. You just had to memorize.

You think about what you are going to do after nursing school. This is pretty much where the Navy came into my life. Navy recruiters came to our school. They just looked so stunning in those dress blue uniforms. There were actually five students who were interested in joining the Navy. I distinctly remember talking to the recruiter. She scheduled a field trip for us to go to Great Lakes Naval Hospital. This

46

hospital was about one hour away. That's really what sealed my decision. She took us around the wards and introduced us to several Navy nurses. I was just bowled over. I was so impressed with their knowledge and professionalism. I learned about the role of the Navy nurse in teaching hospital corpsmen. That pretty much did it for me. I knew I was looking for adventure. I didn't think I was going to find it around Indiana.

My roommate was also interested. We learned about the buddy system. I think, because the two of us could go someplace together, we were brave enough to do this. We were all commissioned at graduation

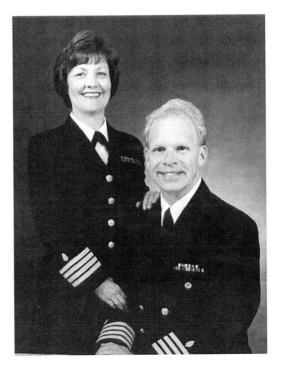

Captain Gloria Caffrey and Captain Jack Caffrey devoted to each other and to the United States of America through service in the United States Navy Nurse Corps. Photo by permission.

from nursing school. We learned very quickly you can ask the Navy anything you want, but you go do what the Navy tells you to do. My roommate and I thought this was our opportunity to go to California. We requested three duty stations in California. We got orders to Philadelphia, Pennsylvania.

I came on active duty in 1970. At this time the Vietnam War was winding down but it was still not a very popular time to be voluntarily joining the military. I had friends who asked me if I was a "warmonger" and would go kill women and children. I had to remove myself from this hate speech and focus on the task at hand: to learn how to be a good Navy nurse and care for the wounded who were just doing the job they were ordered by politicians to do.

I graduated from Depew High School in Depew, New York, in 1963. I did several little jobs after high school: I worked at a steel plant, as a short-order cook and as an orderly at Seneca State School for the mentally disabled in New York State. The cooking job was a disaster. The health department recommended I get into something else. While I was at the State School, I was mentored by one of the first male nurses I ever met, the director of education there. He recommended that I pursue a career in nursing. As an orderly, we had white uniforms and black shoes. The thing that was very cool was that this guy had the same uniform, only he had white shoes. I thought that I would really like to wear white shoes. That led me to ask him about it. He made some inquiries and recommended that I apply to the New York State system for nursing schools that were affiliated with the mental hospitals throughout the state.

Many of the state hospitals had three-year diploma nursing programs subsidized by the state. If you were selected, you got a stipend every month. The goal was to provide professional nurses to staff the system of mental health facilities. I had no intention of staying in psychiatric nursing. My parents couldn't afford college for me. I looked at it as an opportunity to get a good education. My father told me to get a job where there's always going to be job security. My aunt, a registered nurse, told me I couldn't do better than nursing. I thought that was odd because I'm a guy. Nursing is a girl thing. When I was accepted to the three-year program, I found that there were two other men admitted to the same class. Male nurses in this system in 1966 were not unusual, usually constituting about one-third of a class.

I did three years at the Willard State Hospital School of Nursing located in the Finger Lakes region of central of New York. It was a beautiful location. I must say, if you wanted to be crazy, it was the best place to do it. It was an idyllic hospital. When you entered through the main gates, there was a large very old nameplate carved in stone that said, "Willard Hospital for the Insane." Willard was opened in 1842. It was an antique. It was a beautiful place where the patients were very well cared for. There were none of these horror stories that you see.

In my senior year, I made the decision to immediately jump into what New York State called the five-year nursing program. You were coupled onto a state university in a school of nursing. In two years, you got your bachelor's degree. This was very rare. There weren't a lot of BSN nurses around. I figured if I was going to have a successful career, I probably should, while I was in the study mode, just get my BSN out of the way.

I graduated from Willard in 1968 on a Friday. Monday I was in a class at the University of Buffalo School of Nursing. It was called the State University of New York at Buffalo School of Nursing. I was already an RN, because I had passed my boards. In order to make ends meet, I worked in the Veterans Administration Hospital across from the university. I lived at home with my parents, saved money and supported my tuition by working as an RN in the coronary intensive care unit under the guidance of a Franciscan monk. This guy was also an RN and charge nurse of the coronary care unit.

Toward the end of my junior year, I had already received two draft notices. I said to the draft board, "Okay, I'm here. You drafted me." They said, "Well, what are you doing?" I said, "Well, I'm a junior at the University of Buffalo School of Nursing." They said, "Well, that's okay. Go ahead and go back to school. We'll put off your draft until you graduate." I didn't want to just get dumped into the Army. After the second draft notice and they told me to go back to school, I went and started looking for a military career. I figured I was going in the military anyway when I finished. Vietnam was still very hot back then.

I went first to the Air Force. I said, "I am a registered nurse and was wondering if you were accepting male nurses?" The recruiter looked at me and said, "You know we don't take guys in the US Air Force Nurse Corps." I said, "Why is that?" He said, "Well, hell man, you're all queer anyway." I sort of got turned off to the Air Force right then and there. I walked down the hall and bumped into this officer. She was a lieutenant Navy nurse. I told her about my wonderful experience with the Air Force. She said, "Come on in. We'll have a cup of coffee and talk."

She mentioned the Navy Nurse Corps Candidate Program. She said, "If you apply, because you're already an RN, you would be commissioned a year before you graduate. You would be paid as an E3 through your senior year. We'll pay for books and everything. When you graduate with your bachelor's degree, you would come into the Navy and serve three years." I thought, "There you go. I got my bills paid." I made application to the Navy Nurse Corps Candidate Program and was accepted. I was commissioned in October 1969. There were not a lot of male nurses in the Navy at the time, maybe ten. I continued working at the VA, but not nearly as much. I concentrated on my studies and graduated in spring, 1970.

I was given a report date to Newport, Rhode Island, Officer's Indoctrination School in September. I got there and the sign said, "Women's Officer Training School." I thought I was in the wrong place. I showed them my paperwork and said, "If this is the women's officer training, where do us guys go?" They said, "Well, you go here, too, because you're in the nurse corps."

There were three guys, out of one hundred, in our class at Newport. After six weeks, I finished in October. I got my orders to Philadelphia Naval Hospital. I checked in and was assigned to the general medicine *ward under a phenomenal charge nurse. She introduced me to Navy nursing. She was a Vietnam veteran, serving in Da Nang. She had seen a whole lot of action. She was involved in the Tet Offensive. She was a wonderful lieutenant commander and got me on the straight and narrow, setting my feet in the right direction.*

The Vietnam War would last three more years (1973). The Navy established a casualty treatment "pipeline." It started in the field with emergency care, then to "in-country" hospitals or nearby hospital ships where the wounded were triaged and stabilized for evacuation, usually to Okinawa or Guam. At these hospitals, the injured were further treated, prior to being air-evacuated to CONUS. The U.S. military hospitals were designated to treat specific conditions, like orthopedics, neurological injuries, etc. Philadelphia Naval Hospital was designated as a center for ENT, psychiatric conditions, and primarily orthopedics, with a brace and limb department for the amputees. It was also the location for the injured from the East Coast to keep them closer to their homes and family.

The majority of our patients suffered blast injuries (land mines) resulting in internal injuries and amputations. The active-duty personnel were maintained in a medical status until able to be medically discharged from the Navy or returned to active duty. Often that period of rehabilitation could last one or two years. From 1970 to 1972, Philadelphia had an inpatient census of 1,500.

The real heroes of my time in Philadelphia were the Navy hospital corpsmen. These young men and women, most fresh out of high school, needed to be trained in combat casualty care, as they would become the first to render care on the battlefield. Navy nurses had a mission to train the corpsmen as thoroughly as possible to meet that challenge. Often Philadelphia was the first duty station for the male corpsmen to be assigned to Marine Corps units and see heavy fighting and serious injuries. The need for me to do my utmost to train these young men to successfully handle this enormous responsibility became my career focus.

My corpsmen would often relate to certain patients who were severely injured. These patients required intensive nursing care, around the clock monitoring, complicated dressing changes and pain medication. One such patient was a young Marine corporal. He was 21, and suffered blast injuries from stepping on a land mine. He arrived at Philadelphia 72 hours after being injured. He had severe abdominal injuries and amputation of both legs above the knee. He gave the corpsmen experience in colostomy care and complicated stump dressing changes. This Marine was in excellent health prior to his injuries and benefited greatly from the care his corpsmen gave. Over the next two years, this Marine struggled and succeeded in managing his bilateral prosthetic legs, met and eventually married a Navy nurse.

At Philadelphia, I saw the ravages of war, as well as the resilience of young men and women who stepped forward to help our wounded. It was minute by minute teaching these corpsmen to be frontline life savers. Seeing their dedication and eagerness to learn convinced me to focus my career on education, be it hospital corpsmen or any member of the Navy's health care team.

I was in Philly from September 1970 to August 1972. It was a great experience. I worked the first year in medical ICU and decided ICU was not for me. I think the only reason I got to ICU was because I was a three-year grad with lots of clinical experience. There was an opening. There was nobody else on the waiting list. In retrospect, I don't think it was such a great idea. We had cardiac monitors, but they were all bedside monitors. You had to walk around and look for irregular rhythms. It was just a big open ICU. After ICU, I went back to the medicine wards.

My first supervisor was infamous. I really have to credit her for me staying in the Navy. My intention was to fulfill my obligations and get out. She was one tough supervisor in a good way. Right at the onset, she instilled the importance of teaching the corpsmen everything that we could. In the '70s, Vietnam was still going on. She said, "You're not going to go to the front, but your corpsmen will. You'd better make sure they have every tool in their bag that you can possibly give them." I think she really gave all of us a real sense of purpose as to what it meant to be in the nurse corps. Your responsibilities for teaching corpsmen were unlike any civilian nursing job. Looking back, I think I reported to Philadelphia as a "nurse in the Navy." When I left, I was a "Navy nurse."

I started out in general medicine. We had very interesting cases. Probably 98 percent of them were Vietnam connected. We also had a contingent of Veterans Administration Beneficiaries (VAB). They were overflow from the Philadelphia Veterans Administration Hospital. I was one of the few with a bachelor's degree.

I was right around the corner from the ICU. I would receive a lot of patients from the ICU to my ward. It was a forty-bed open ward. One day, I got a patient transfer from the ICU. This cute little ensign brought him over and introduced herself. She said, "Hi, my name is Ensign Gloria Huitsing." She was from a little town called Highland, Indiana. We just sort of said hi and transferred the patient.

When I got to the wards, I had more opportunity to work with active duty, particularly on ENT and lower GI surgery wards. It was funny because Jack was the charge nurse on 2C. He got transferred to nursing education. I took over as the charge nurse of that ward. One thing I remember is how much the patients helped each other. That's when you had a ward master-at-arms (MAA). Patients actually did a lot of the work. They took care of each other. Over the years, that went away when outside cleaning services were contracted, and with the introduction of private and semi-private rooms. The patients couldn't see the guy in the next bed, so what was happening with him didn't impact others. This idea has come full-circle now in the rehab units that have opened up in Camp Lejeune and Camp Pendleton. In those two hospitals, the patients, the Marines, are back helping each other. Another thing I recall is how much the corpsmen helped the patients outside of work. It was common for corpsmen to take patients, who could go on liberty, over to the sports stadium across the street from the hospital. Professional sports teams would donate tickets and the guys would go have a blast. I don't think it mattered what teams were playing. It was good therapy for the patients to go out and do normal things.

The other thing I remember about Philly is that it really helped me get organized because of the way we had to cover the PM and the night shifts. When you worked days, you were on one unit. In my area, for PMs, we had to cover two wards. On nights we had to cover four wards. We had pockets full of all the keys we had to carry for all the narcotic lockers. In our units, we would draw up the pre-ops and just put the syringes on the med cart and say to the corpsmen, "Okay, just give this at 6:00 a.m.," and then we'd leave. I remember on PMs one night, I went into the solarium. It sure smelled pretty sweet in there. I knew they were smoking a few joints. I never caught anybody, but you could smell it. I remember one night I covered two of the orthopedic wards. Instead of four wards, I had six wards to cover. I got through it. I didn't kill anybody, and learned a lot.

I met my husband, Jack, at Philly. Jack got orders to Great Lakes Naval Hospital to the Hospital Corps School. The chief nurse asked me, "Your obligation is coming to an end. Have you thought about what you want to do?" I said, "Well, I'm pretty happy in the Navy. I really like what I'm doing. I see a lot of opportunity, etc." She said, "Would you like to go to Great Lakes?" I said, "That would be wonderful. My family is 75 miles from Great Lakes and that would give me an opportunity to see my family more often." Then she smiled with a little twinkle in her eye and said, "Well, isn't there another reason you'd like to go to Great Lakes?" She was a matchmaker. She had already arranged it. She had called the detailer. The detailer said, "Yes, we can send her to the Great Lakes Naval Hospital." The chief nurse was a wonderful person, especially to the junior officers (JOs). She told the supervisors, when filling out the schedules, she wanted every nurse, including the JOs, to have every other weekend off. If they couldn't figure out the schedules and how to make that happen, they needed to bring their schedules to the nursing office. She would help them figure out how to do that. There was no supervisor that was going to do that. I never worked two weekends in a row. It was hard enough for us to do the night/PMs/day rotations. Now we know if you have to rotate shifts, that is not the way to do it. We all did it.

During my time in Philadelphia, we were told to be very discreet about where we wore uniforms off base. We could travel to and from the hospital in uniform, but no stopping for gas or groceries, etc. Best to not advertise your active-duty status for fear of ridicule or attack by an angry public. Unlike in more recent times, none was going to thank you for your service or buy you lunch.

I got involved in the Junior Nurse Corps Association. In short order, I was elected as president. I hated the way we administered medication. Every night the night corpsmen had to write down all the medications for each patient in their chart for every dose they would receive the next day. That was the routine every night. In my off hours I sat down and created a form and called it the Medication Administration Record (MAR). I presented it to my charge nurse and supervisor. This form provided a way to do the same job on a month-long basis. We kept patients for a long time then. I wrote up the instructions on how it was to be used. The chief nurse called me down to the office. She said, "You know, I've looked at your form. I think it has potential. I would like to pursue getting it approved for test here at Philadelphia." I said, "Yes, ma'am, I'd be happy to do whatever I can to help out." She got permission from BUMED in D.C. to trial test the form. Our Junior Nurse Corps Association was charged with conducting the study. We made very few modifications to the original. Before I left Philadelphia, the chief nurse notified me that the Bureau of Medicine and Surgery had accepted my MAR for distribution and use throughout the Navy. That was the highlight of Philly.

While at Philadelphia, Gloria and I started dating. We were extremely discreet. When we went on dates it was when we could arrange to get together with our time schedules. She was in the previous class at Newport. She had about a month and a half ahead of me on station. We were both getting ready for orders. Because I had done so much training at the hospital to teach the staff how to use the MAR, the chief nurse

called me down and said, "How would you like to go teach corps school?"
I said, "Well, I probably prefer to go to Vietnam and get that taken care
of." She said, "Well, we really need people qualified to teach at corps
school. You are one of the few here who has a bachelor's degree. That's
very important, so where would you like to go, Great Lakes, Illinois, or
San Diego, California?" I had never been to California. I said, "I would
love to go to California." She said, "Okay fine, get out of here."

She talked to the detailers and called me back to the office maybe
a half hour later. She said, "Well, I've got your orders to corps school." I
said, "Oh great, California sun." She said, "No, you're going to go to Great
Lakes." I thought "Oh gee. Here Glo and I have been dating a little over a
year and what's this going to do?" I went to leave and then I stopped and
said, "Excuse me, Captain, I have an issue going on." She said, "Are you
kidding, everybody in the hospital knows about your little issue. Don't
worry, Gloria will be following you by one month. She will be stationed in
Naval Hospital Great Lakes." All the time, all the supervisors, the chief
and assistant chief nurse knew we were dating. We wanted to be discreet.
We were brand new to the Navy. We thought we needed to be the best offi-
cers we could. We thought we had to be careful, but everybody knew.

From 1972 to 1976, I was at Great Lakes Naval Hospital. I started
out on a female medical-surgical floor. I worked there for about three
months. This was dependents med-surg, private and semi-private
rooms. In Philly, if you counted all the in-patients, the ramps with all
the psych patients and all the ortho patients, there were 1,500 patients.
Great Lakes had a couple hundred patients, so much smaller. My ward
had maybe 30. I didn't like that ward so much. I had nothing against
female patients, but I really wanted to care for male patients, in particular active-duty male patients.

A friend of mine worked in the OR and said, "Why don't you come
and work in the operating room? Why don't you come down someday, see what we do and talk to the supervisor?" My chief nurse said,
"Yes, you can come work in the OR, but we have a shortage in labor
and delivery for a month. Even though you've never worked labor and
delivery and you have no experience, you're going to go work in labor
and delivery for a while." I figured that was my time in hell before the
OR. It didn't matter whether you had any experience, you just went and
did what you were told. So, I did my time in labor and delivery. I didn't
deliver any babies there. I was on two weeks of days to get me oriented.
Then, they put me on nights and PMs by myself. I had every OB complication patient you could think of, no normal deliveries. I will never
step in labor and delivery again. It was pretty scary. I had patients with

prolapsed cords, abruptio placenta, C-sections because patients couldn't deliver, eclampsia, seizures, you name it. I would call the supervisor. A lot of time, that didn't help. The supervisor couldn't help me. The doctors were absolutely wonderful. I probably learned more from them in a couple of weeks than anybody. They knew the situation. They didn't leave the patient. They were excellent. It taught me a lot about what to look for, but it still was a pretty frightening experience.

I went down to the OR and that's where I really found my niche. I didn't think I was going to like it as much as I did. I fell in love with it. I couldn't wait to go to work. I was so excited about all the different things that happened in the OR and the things I was learning. Working in an OR requires a lot of planning and organization. I think I am naturally a pretty organized person, but the Philadelphia experiences, especially covering all those wards on nights, really helped me to adapt to the OR.

I had a couple of very wonderful OR supervisors there. There are significant people in your past that are great mentors and role models and those two, in particular, were mine for the OR. Sadly, these two nurses have passed from different types of cancers. One was stationed at the Da Nang Field Hospital and the other on the hospital ship, where they cared for patients directly from combat. I can't help but wonder if their cancers (and those of many other Navy nurses who have passed) were related to coming in contact with Agent Orange chemicals on the clothing of the injured.

I relate the following stories to the best of my ability: The nurse who was at Da Nang told me about the grueling hours, how she dreaded the "whop, whop" sound of the helicopters coming in with casualties, and how she could never get the blood stains out of her shoelaces. How one night, there were several head injuries and the one neurosurgeon operated two days straight. She held up his arms so he could keep operating. The nurse on the hospital ship told me about the first time she pulled duty on the flight deck with incoming casualties. She was used to getting patients in the OR, all prepped for surgery, but not accustomed to seeing them directly from the battlefield. She freaked. After her first shift, she left sobbing and told the medical officer in charge that she couldn't work there again. He told her she would indeed work there again. "You will put on a clean uniform, makeup, and perfume, because you are the best thing that Marine (who just lost a leg) has seen in months." It was not about her ... it was about the patients. I miss these two nurses so much, such a wealth of experience, such wonderful friendships, gone too soon.

At Great Lakes, we did have the opportunity to care for some of the Vietnam POWs because their families were in the Chicago area. A couple of them needed some surgery for untreated injuries like bones that had been broken and needed to be reset. It was an honor to care for these men who had endured so much, yet were thankful for the care they were given by the staff at Great Lakes.

While I was at Great Lakes, my supervisor said, "Gloria, if you want to stay in the Navy, a diploma nurse is fine, but the Navy expects more. You really need to think about finishing up your requirements for your bachelor's degree." I went to school part-time at the community college, working on the credits that I needed. I applied for DUINS (duty under instruction) and got accepted. From 1976 to 1978, I was DUINS at Medical University of South Carolina (MUSC) in Charleston. I chose this university because we were married. I looked for schools near duty stations where Jack and I could be together.

I got orders to Great Lakes. I was assigned as an instructor at the Hospital Corps School. I was one of four guys there. Apparently, they planted a lot of the guys in corps school. The men that came into the US Navy Nurse Corps during that period also had bachelor's degrees. I thought that was unusual. There wasn't a two-year program back then. There was only a three-year diploma and baccalaureate programs. Many of the male nurses were former corpsmen and knew where the education had to be. They subsequently got out, went to school, and came back in. One of the guys there went on to be a commanding officer for three commands. He was just a phenomenal mentor for me. I spent the rest of the next four years as a division officer, teaching Hospital Corps School. We didn't have women coming through at the time. I think they were trained someplace else. I loved the tour. I loved teaching. It really was my niche. I hated leaving corps school, but left in 1976. I was having a great time. I got 4.0 fit reps while I was there. I also oriented all the new instructors that came in. I guess I was just doing a great job, so they just kept me there. It wasn't like we were short of instructors. I don't know why, but I just had an extraordinarily long tour at Corps School.

Half way through my corps school tour, Glo and I got married. We had a military wedding with the swords and side boys. I was in military uniform. She wore her wedding gown. It was a great military wedding. We were married at the Navy chapel at the Naval Training Center at Great Lakes in 1974.

By that time, we were senior lieutenants. We started doing our own research on how to best stay together. We started talking to the detailers in more depth, trying to learn the billet structures, the education and experience requirements needed for certain types of jobs. We went looking for our own billets in order to stay together.

I requested a billet at the Naval Hospital Charleston in the nursing education department because they had an opening. I got it. The trick that we figured out was to find out what the Navy needs, compare it to what we like, and come up with a happy medium. We did that for the rest of our careers. I was selected for the billet in nursing education at the hospital. We started our two-year tour at Charleston. I worked as an instructor in the nursing education department and did PM and night supervision.

When I checked into Charleston, it was really weird. I checked in with another nurse, a female nurse. We checked in to see the chief nurse the same day. The secretary said to her, "You can go in and meet the chief nurse." She finished up and left. I'm still sitting there. The secretary said, "Lieutenant, what are you doing here?" I said, "Well, I just checked in and I'm supposed to meet with the captain." She said, "But the captain never greets new male nurses, only the female nurses." I said, "You're kidding me?" She said, "No, that's the way it's done. She just does not like or talk to the male nurses." I said, "Well, today's the last day of that habit. I'm going in." I knocked on her door. She said, "Who's there?" I said, "Good morning," I introduced myself and said, "Can I come in and give you a brief on my experience?" She was shocked. She was visibly shaking. She couldn't handle a guy. She obviously couldn't handle men in the profession. I was in there for an hour. We wound up friends over time. She was an absolutely amazing lady and we got along very well. I did several special projects for her. I remember her sending me a letter after her retirement thanking me for breaking that tradition of hers.

In some respects, school was a little difficult. I found some of the faculty were a little demeaning to the RN students. I found that we were not always respected for what we knew. I found the clinical sometimes to be difficult. I was used to doing what Navy nurses do. I was used to being in charge. I had to remind myself that the nurse aides were not corpsmen. I got through it.

Again, I just sort of got bitten by the education bug. I applied for a Ph.D. program in DUINS. I got two master's degrees while I was in Charleston. Because I worked regular hours, I was able to go to school at night. Webster University had a campus at the Air Force base at Charleston. I would go over there and attend classes. I got a dual master's in communication and health care administration, and an MBA. I applied for a Ph.D. program in nursing education through the DUINS program. I applied to George Washington University and several other places. I got accepted to all those universities. They were all local because we figured if we stayed in the D.C. area, Glo could do her thing.

After school we had our only separation. We had orders to Rota, Spain. I had to go right after I graduated from school in June. Because of funding, Jack couldn't go until October. We had a four-month separation. That's the longest one we ever had. It would have been easy if it had been Stateside, but overseas was a little difficult. I lived in the BOQ for the first three months or so. I had plenty of time to go out and find us a place to live. We decided we did not want to live on base. That's not why we went to Spain. I had the time and the luxury to find a place where I knew we could be happy. I actually found the house. Jack was packing up and the furniture was being loaded back in South Carolina. At the last minute I called him and said, "Don't put that big furniture on the truck. That house is small. It's never going to hold all our furniture." At the last minute, the movers were pulling things off the truck and putting it in storage.

We were the first married nurse corps couple that was sent overseas. We kind of had to fight to get overseas orders. It hadn't been done before so, "How's it going to work?" and "It's a small duty station," were some of the questions the nurse corps was asking. We just said, "We'll make it work." It was a small duty station. We had 22 nurses at that hospital. We all worked different shifts. The hospital had a military ward, dependent ward, two bed ICU, delivery room, nursery, two operating rooms, an ER and out-patient clinics. I was detailed as a general staff nurse. The hospital already had an OR nurse. I relieved in the OR but mostly worked as a staff nurse. We worked both sides of the wards, the ER, and the clinics. Everybody had to learn how to cover the OR. Everybody had to learn how to do an appendectomy and a C-section. I helped train them.

One of the fun things about Rota was the contact with the fleet. The ships came in and the active-duty sailors were there. One thing that used to drive us nuts, but about which we certainly had a great understanding, was the psychiatric patients that were dropped off from the ship. Believe it or not, in the hospital our sickest patients were often the psych patients. Many of them had to be medevacked back to the States. Sometimes, that medevac system worked too slowly. I remember one patient who was in four-point restraints secondary to being suicidal for about three weeks waiting to be transferred. I just thought that was unacceptable.

On the plus side of the medevac system, we got to hop on it sometimes and go somewhere. Jack and I only took one big hop. You had to plan your leave in advance. With only 22 nurses, only two nurses could be gone at one time. We took the medevac up to Germany, the train for a week in Holland, the train back to Germany and spent a week in the Garmisch area of the Alps. It was a long leave, but everybody took their turn. In Rota, we would all wait for the new shipment of Lladros. The exchange had a great contract with the factory. We needed to get a Lladro vase appraised once. We had two of them and I was going to put one of them in an auction. The appraiser found that a lot of the Lladros that we bought were never sent to the United States. It was appraised at $500. I bought it for $30.

Jack and I both made lieutenant commander in Rota. That was kind of a big event. I remember probably the worst night of my Navy career. I was working the PM shift. In Spain, people drove around in little, tiny cars with ten people in them. One of our family practice doctors was in one of those little cars with his wife, their three children, another couple, and their two children. They were hit by a train because many of the trains did not have crossing guards. He, his wife and one son of the other couple survived. The rest were killed. That was a terrible night. He and his wife came into our hospital. He was very badly injured and had to be medevacked. She was, amazingly, not injured at all, but was hysterical. It was a very difficult night knowing what had happened to the family.

We took our Great Dane, Eric, with us to Spain. He was only about two years old when we left Charleston. We decided we couldn't leave him, so we took him to Spain with us. When Jack came to Spain, he flew commercial because he had the dog and a military plane couldn't accommodate him. I think he had to pay a nominal fee for the dog, but no extra fee for himself. During the whole three years we were there, we were one of the few American couples living off base that weren't robbed. We attribute that to the dog. When we went to work in the morning, we made sure the blinds were open. The dog was so intimidating, the Spanish in our neighborhood used to call him "little horse." How he loved to run on the beach and scare the natives!!

Just before I went to Spain, my father passed away. That made the transition difficult. If you had a death in the family, they made every effort to get you back to the States, especially active-duty officers. After the funeral, Glo went back to Spain. I went back to Charleston and finished up my real-estate issues.

Rota only had billets for general nursing. I started out as a staff nurse and did orientation for incoming nurses. I performed a myriad of tasks from Rota: charge nurse for the out-patient department, instructor for CPR and CPR instructors, coordinator and lead instructor for CPR instruction, training and certifying all CPR instructors in all Navy facilities in Europe, CPR training for flight line crews.

Three great years in Spain had to come to an end. From 1981 to 1985 we were at Bethesda. I went directly to the OR. It really was a shock coming from a small duty station back to a place like Bethesda. Everything was a shock: the workload, the commute, the shortage of OR nurses. In the OR we had a terrible shortage of nurses, horrendous hours, plus a difficult political environment. When we went to Bethesda, I was already programmed to go to the Naval School of Health Sciences (NSHS) to head up the OR technician school. For the one year I was in the OR at Bethesda, I "floated."

I have great appreciation for anybody who, by choice, is a floater. It is a really tough thing to do. You have to be knowledgeable about all these different surgical services. Usually in the OR, you get assigned consistently to two specific services. If you float, you're in all of the different services all of the time. I did it intentionally. I knew I was going to the school. I had been out of the OR for a while. I needed to brush up on everything. I'm glad I did it, but it certainly wasn't easy.

I was at NSHS for three years. Once again, I found myself in another teaching role, but this time the corpsmen had been screened for advanced training as surgical technicians in the OR. There were four enlisted instructors and me. It was so gratifying to watch our students progress from nervous novices to competent scrub technicians, capable of handling the most complex surgical cases.

During this time there were a lot of issues in operating rooms. Some of the situations were leadership issues with the nurses and the supervisors. The Nurse Corps decided that maybe it was time to let some OR nurses go back for master's degrees. It was not a group that had been targeted before. My CO said, "You should apply for this. I'll give you a really good recommendation." I said, "Well, I've already been DUINS once for my bachelor's degree." "It doesn't matter. Go ahead and write up your application." She gave me this glowing endorsement. I was accepted.

Big facilities, like Bethesda, could absorb us. I was assigned as a clinical instructor. I worked in medicine, surgery, oncology and neurology. I was covering four services as a clinical instructor. I oriented all new nurses and corpsmen. I did PM and night supervision. There were times the United States president was in-house. I got to meet some interesting people. Arleigh Burke, for whom the Burke Class destroyers were named, was one.

From 1985 to 1987 we were back in the Chicago area. I was at DePaul University in Chicago for my master's degree. I spent two more years in school. The students all had a lot of experience. The faculty was very respectful of that. I think the DUINS is one of the best gifts the Navy ever gave me. My degree was in nursing administration with a focus in operating room management. For any projects, papers, I would try to find an OR related topic. I knew I would be going back to an OR after the master's program. However, the seed was planted by my faculty. For the first time ever, I thought seriously that I could be a director of nursing. I put it on my goal list down the road.

The chief nurse of Bethesda called me down and said, "I want you to take this phone call." She left the room and shut the door. The person on the phone said, "This is the admiral and director of the United States Navy Nurse Corps. I am currently in the DUINS selection board. We have a situation here. Because of our billet end strength, we are not capable of selecting a Ph.D. candidate this year. Otherwise, we would select you. However, the Navy line has asked us to initiate a new program called Education and Training Management at George Washington University. It's a twelve-month master's program. It is extremely expensive. You will be the first Navy nurse to go to this program, if you accept this instead of your doctorate program. If you don't accept this new program, we can't select you. If you accept, we can select you for a brand-new sub-designator for the nurse corps. You will actually get the M.Ed. from GW." I said, "Hell, Admiral, I would be happy to." That was what qualified me for a doctorate. We had never sent anyone for a master's in education management. The admiral was a proponent for establishing a separate BUMED position, which would become the Bureau of Medical Education Management.

I completed that program and was due for orders. What do you do with this guy who has this unique master's degree that the Navy Nurse Corps wants to showcase? There were now geographical commands that covered the big sections of the country, Great Lakes, Jacksonville, and San Diego. The Great Lakes command managed everything from Chicago east, all the Navy hospitals and facilities in the Northeast. Jacksonville covered all the Navy facilities in the Southeast, and San Diego had the whole West Coast. The director said, "I'm establishing a position for each one of these Geo-Coms for education and training. You are going to be the first one to man one of those billets coming out of graduate school."

In 1985, I got orders to the Navy Medical Command Northeast Region (GEO-COM) in Great Lakes, Illinois. I managed, coordinated and standardized education for nursing, all enlisted hospital corps, medicine and dentistry throughout the Northeast. I had to learn about continuing education, DUINS programs and upward mobility programs for the enlisted. We did a tremendous amount of traveling. Because I was one of the few people with a background in education in large medical facilities, I got tapped to do a lot of Navy medical IG, naval hospital IG inspections, augmentee work, and BCLS (basic life support). I did this for two years. During this time, we both made commander.

From 1987 to 1991 we were stationed in Jacksonville, Florida. We decided it was finally time for some warmer weather. We experienced Bethesda with a couple of killer blizzards and six years in Great Lakes. That's a lot of winter. We thought it was time to go to Florida. I was the department head of the OR. Again, the OR nurse shortage was still on-going. Even though I was the department head, many days I had to staff a room and take calls, just like everybody else.

Jacksonville was my first time in the south. We found the Jacksonville community to be one of the most proud and supportive Navy-friendly areas we had lived in. I was assigned as the education and training coordinator for the GEO command in the Southeast. We bought a house down there and sort of got settled. For the next two years, I essentially did the same thing I did up in Great Lakes, only for the Southeast. We got to Jacksonville in 1987, but in 1989, the Geo-Com concept died. I was unemployed. In 1989, they gave me orders to the hospital. I thought, "Okay, fine. I'll go work in education over there and do my thing." I walked in and the CO said, "Well, the nursing education department is fine. We don't need you there." I thought I was going to be cleaning floors. He said, "You're going to be my special assistant. You're going to be my point man and coordinator for the preparation of the Navy IG."

The hospital was in bad shape, outside of its nursing education department. I knew about the Navy IG (inspector general). I knew the criteria. I knew the hospital wasn't going to pass. They were in terrible shape. It was because of a long list of difficulties and poor management on the part of a string of COs and department heads. It was really probably the low point of my career. He gave me all the responsibility to pull together this command and none of the authority. It made it nearly impossible.

For almost a year, I was responsible for bringing this command back to where it needed to be. I gave the CO all kinds of regular reports, telling him who was not compliant. About four months before the IG, I said, "You're going to fail and this is where you're going to fail." I gave him a complete report on every department in the command, where they were not compliant and everything I had done to try and change it. He said, "Well, I'll just file this." The IG came and sat down with me. They all knew me. They did a complete evaluation of the facility. Essentially, their out-going report was a carbon copy of what I had given four months earlier. The hospital flunked inspection. I got an award. I think it was a Navy Commendation for what I did. It wasn't the outcome one would expect, but it was a very unusual situation.

Toward the very end of our tour in 1991, the director of Nursing Service called me and said, "You and Gloria are both in the zone for captain. This will be the first time a married couple will be considered for 06 in the same board, at the same time. It will be interesting to see what they will come up with." The board results came out. We got a call to come down to the commanding officer's office. I thought, "Oh no, which-ever one of us does not make captain is going to get out of the Navy." We came down and everybody started applauding. We were both selected at the same board for captain. Sadly, it meant we had to have orders.

We were told we had to go back to Bethesda. I was assigned as the associate director of nursing for preoperative services. This time, for me, it was different. Now, it was all of the politics that go on at the senior levels. The OR nursing shortage was continuing. This time, I had a chance to do something about it. I was also assigned as a specialty advisor for peri-operative nursing. Every clinical specialty in the Navy Medical Department: medical, nursing, dental, allied health and administrative, has a specialty advisor to the surgeon general to bring issues to the forefront. Also, when there are JAG reviews for litigation cases, they need expert advice to review those cases. My first week at Bethesda, I was welcomed with two of these JAG cases that have to be reviewed. I had a situation in the heart room of incorrect sponge count recorded as correct. The patient had to be brought back to the OR. Not enough staff, too many surgeons, an admiral telling me how to staff the OR to get more "bang for the buck." I thought, "Oh, wait a minute. What did I walk into?"

Because I was a specialty advisor, I was able to write some position papers to give to the nurse corps admiral recommendations to fix the shortage. We converted some general duty nurse positions to OR nurse positions. We were able to get civil service positions in the OR for the first time. We were able to recall reservists for one, two, three-year assignments to staff the OR. We set up a selection board process and established qualifications, so that nurses who wanted to transfer to the OR were screened and qualified. I had a lot of support, especially from the doctors and the chief of surgery. He knew the more he supported me, the more it would help his surgeons and their training programs.

I think that was why I was sent to Bethesda, though I didn't want to go. I did it kicking and screaming. Sometimes you see a problem and you say, "Boy, I'm going to do something about that when I'm senior and have a chance." That's probably one of the things that I'm most proud of in my career. I talked to nurses all the time that wanted to be in the OR, but there weren't any openings. There were no billets because there weren't *enough* billets. We did a top-down review of all the naval hospitals. We looked at the number of ORs, how many cases and shifts they ran, how many nurses they had, how they scheduled, what would they do if they had more, etc. We got surveys from all of our naval hospitals. The data was just unquestionable. That's how we got our OR staffed, in the long run. It's a really good thing we did. The up tempo in the Middle East since Desert Shield–Desert Storm, then Iraq and Afghanistan, made it important to have better staffed operating rooms. I think the payoff lasts for a long time.

After four years at Bethesda, Jack and I are chomping at the bit to come back to Jacksonville. Once you're a senior officer, you do a decent job and you get to the Washington, D.C., area, they never want to let you go. In 1995, we thought we were going to go back to Jacksonville. That didn't happen. From 1995 to 1998 I was assigned to BUPERS (Bureau of Personnel) as the senior nurse corps detailer/assignment officer. I thought, why not. If it isn't me, it will be somebody else and I will have to deal with them. I loved that job. It was totally a different kind of assignment and command, not medical. The job was not just saying, "Okay, you're going to go here or there." It was lot of career-shaping and career counseling. There were some unhappy people. There were times I thought I would go out to the parking lot and find my tires slashed. There are a lot of times I'd say to somebody, "You haven't been overseas. You need to go to Guam or Okinawa." A lot of them didn't want to go, but it was not uncommon for me to get an email message from someone six months to a year later saying, "Thank you for sending me here. It's been a great experience."

I talked with the director and deputy director of the Navy Nurse Corps. I said, "You know I think it's time for a little bit more transparency in the detailing process. It is time to de-mystify what goes on here and to eliminate the idea of favoritism." That was the perception, true or untrue. We did a lot of detailing traveling and visits. We posted the billets that were open so somebody could go on line to see what billets were available. It wasn't like we held anything in secret. Still people didn't always get what they wanted, but, had a sense that they could try. There wasn't something that was being held open for a friend who was very popular. It was really exciting to be able to work with the leadership of the nurse corps to shape the corps for the future. I was at BUPERS for three years. Added to the four years at Bethesda, it was seven years in D.C. that we hadn't planned on.

At Bethesda, I started working in nursing education at Health Sciences Education & Training Command (HSETC), running the DUINS program for nurses, Navy wide. I was also responsible for overseeing the Medical Enlisted Commission Education Program, selecting enlisted persons for nursing and health care degrees. The first year the nurse corps admiral said, "I want you to start up the nurse corps executive conferences." That was a worldwide conference of all senior Navy nurses coming to Washington for a five-day conference. It hadn't been done before. It was a huge, huge thing for the nurse corps. I was in charge of putting together three of these conferences.

For the second conference in 1992, we needed a keynote speaker. I said, "Why don't we invite Hillary Rodham Clinton?" The admiral looked at me and said, "There isn't any way that's going to happen, not in this world of politics. Besides the Clintons are pushing healthcare reform. We're not big enough in the big scheme of things to attract her attention." I said, "Well, I think we are." You wouldn't believe what kind of chop-chain is involved in order to get an invitation to the White House, in addition to setting up this huge Nurse Corps Executive Conference. As things turned out we had a phenomenal meeting. It was topped off by our keynote speaker, Hillary Rodham Clinton. She was super. It was not the nurse corps conferences that I ran, but the nurses I got to know. I felt and saw those who applied for, got and went through the DUINS program in the three years I had the job. It was those kids I now see retire as captains after very successful careers. That was the greatest part of that tour being the director of Nurse Corps Education.

After that tour I did the DUINS selection board every year. There was an opening for XO at HSETC and I was selected in 1997. We did some reorganization and managed a budget of more than 50 million dollars a year. Then, I was selected as commanding officer and moved across the hall. They asked me if I wanted to stay for a full command tour of three years. I told them no. I preferred to leave D.C. and get back to Jacksonville, where Glo and I wanted to retire. I had 28 years by then.

It was a happy day when I wrote the orders to myself and Jack to go back to Jacksonville. Jack always joked that he got orders back to Jacksonville because he slept with the detailer. From 1998 to 2000, we were back in Jacksonville.

At Jacksonville I was assigned as the senior nurse executive/director of nursing service. This is my chance to be the chief nurse. I've waited 28 years for this position, only to find that they have done this major product line reorganization. I found that almost all of the nurses didn't report to me. They report to their product line director. However, as director of nursing service, I'm still responsible for the nursing care that is provided by the nurses that don't report to me. They did this major reorganization and then left. They never really had to work with it. It was in place when I got there. I could see that it was not going to change. I figured I'd better make the most of it.

What I had to do was find a way to establish a connection with the nurses. We reviewed all the nursing care and the standards. All the fitness reports of the nurses came through me. I was also responsible for all of the career counseling. I would say that probably my experiences in the detailing office really helped me figure out how to make this dysfunctional organization work. It was a bit disappointing. It was not what I expected. I could find ways to have the influence, but the control was difficult. It was not uncommon to meet with a junior officer and have them say to me, "I don't work for you," which technically was true.

I had the good fortune to marry a very smart woman who was also the senior detailer. She has been my wife for 30 some years. We found billets available in Jacksonville, her as the director of nursing and me as an open 2900 billet. One of the prettiest pictures we had ever seen was Washington, D.C., in the rearview mirror. We had spent 11 years of our 30 in Washington.

We moved back to our original home in Jacksonville and checked in at the hospital. I met with the commanding officer of the hospital. He wanted me to stand in for him whenever he had to be out of town. My assignment was director of operational medicine. That was the management of all of the branch medical clinics in Georgia and Florida, from Athens, outside of Atlanta, down to Key West. My responsibilities included coordinating all the ambulatory care in the branch clinics. These included a very large sub base clinic at King's Bay Naval Station, Mayport Clinic for carriers, clinics at NAS Jacksonville, Orlando and Key West. One of the jobs I was doing was to coordinate military construction and deconstruction. We closed the clinic in Orlando and Cecil Field, and began construction for brand new clinics in Athens, Mayport and Key West. That was one of the many projects I had to do. It kept me very busy for the last two years of our tour.

In looking back, I'm disappointed that I did not have an operational tour. I would have loved to have gone on a ship. When I was a lieutenant, a lot of my male OR nurse colleagues would get orders to the ships. I thought, "I'm a better OR nurse than they are. I'm more organized than they are." It was very frustrating to see them go and know that the only reason I couldn't go was because I was a female. When Desert Storm came around, I was the OR department head in Jacksonville. I told my boss I would go. But, our CO made the decision that no department heads would be deployed. He said, "It's easier to send a staff nurse out and get a staff nurse in than it is to lose my department heads." It made sense. I wasn't deployed during Desert Storm because of the position I had. Even though I had a wonderful 30-year career, it personally was disappointing to me that I never had a deployment.

Jack and I retired together on May 3, 2000, in a joint ceremony.

If you fail to select for flag and you reach the three-year mark and you're on active duty, it meant retirement. This was fine because you get a good chunk of your active duty pay. We started planning our retirement ceremony. We had it just outside the Navy hospital. By that time, we had a new commanding officer. The XO was the current surgeon general. The keynote speaker was a former director of the Navy Nurse Corps. I am told we were the first married couple in the Navy to complete 30 years together. I know that there was a married couple in the reserve line who were both admirals. As far as nursing was concerned, we were the only ones. We had a very nice retirement ceremony.

Jack and I were fortunate to have such good careers and be able to be stationed together. We made some compromises along the way trying to work out assignments. Our duty stations were all good in different ways. If you asked us if we would do it all over again, the answer would be an emphatic "YES!" It was the Philadelphia experience that laid the groundwork for two 30 year careers, for lifelong friendships, and for two people who tried to make a difference as "Navy nurses."

Elaine J. Dlouhy

I GRADUATED FROM Farragut High School in Chicago, Illinois, in 1956. I knew I wanted to be a nurse. My older sister was a nurse and I idolized her. The least expensive way to achieve that goal was a diploma school of nursing in Chicago, Michael Reese Hospital School of Nursing. A young lady could get an education and have a marketable skill the rest of her life. At 17 years of age, I went to nursing school.

I was always a very goal-oriented child. Nothing was going to stand in my way. I did very well in nursing school, academically. I did well, not super, in regard to clinical. We did not get any administration experience. We were excellent bedside nurses. I've noticed, in later years looking back, some of us have it and some of us don't, in terms of becoming a leader. There were times in school when we were scared to death because we were the only nurse on a busy surgical ward. We had a nurse's aide to help us with 25 or more patients. There was no post-op area, and very little time in recovery. There was nothing like an ICU. People stayed in hospitals longer then. Of course, there weren't all these fancy machines to learn about. People died more often. There were fewer medications. I realized how stressful it was. Now, when my classmates and I get together, we kind of laugh about it. I think I got through school with flying colors.

My father died, leaving an inheritance of $2,000 for me to go back to school to get a bachelor's degree. With the inheritance money and the help of my mother, who continued working, I got through school. I had already saved money through high school. My mother was not pro-education, but she always saw to it I had the physical things I needed. She was really very kind. Between my frugality and my mother's generosity, I did well through school, as far as money went.

My choice was the University of Illinois. I always wanted to go to a big college campus. I finally had the wonderful experience of being on a college campus. It is something you lack at a diploma school of nursing, where you work 44 hours a week, including classes. It wasn't

68

easy. They didn't know what to do with students who were already registered nurses. There were about six that started the same time I did. I didn't meet them until we got to our extended clinical at Illinois Research Hospital in Chicago. While I was at the University of Illinois Medical Center campus, I worked weekends at Mount Sinai Hospital, also in Chicago.

We had to repeat some of our diploma school courses. They wanted us to take nutrition, anatomy, physiology, and leadership all over again. It ended up being three semesters at the university campus and four quarters at

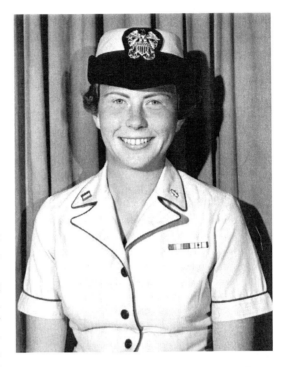

Lieutenant Elaine Dlouhy, March 1968. Elaine was very goal oriented from becoming a registered nurse to maturing as a Navy Nurse Corps officer. Photo by permission.

the medical center campus. I had already taken state boards after the diploma program, but they made us take the NLN graduate nurse qualifying exam. It is like taking state boards over again. They didn't make it easy for us to get that degree. I was very glad I got it before I joined the Navy.

I worked a total of seven years as a civilian, starting at the Illinois State Psychiatric Institute. I later went back to Mount Sinai Hospital in Chicago and taught nursing skills to their student nurses. At a military orientation class for seniors while I was teaching there, three recruiters came to tell them about nursing in the military. The Navy nurse recruiter happened to be a graduate from my school of nursing in Chicago and recognized my pin and cap. She cornered me and said, "Have you thought about joining the military?" I had thought about it. I was soon to be 26 years old. I did not have a boyfriend and was concerned about how I was going to take care of myself the rest of my life. I did not like staying in the same hospital forever. I knew in the military

I could move around. I enjoyed traveling already. I knew there would be an exchange of people. You didn't have to wait until somebody died. She encouraged me to join.

The sister I mentioned earlier had married an Army man. He was a career artilleryman. He said, "Elaine, if you're going to join the military, you'd better do it now. You're going to be at an age when you're going to be ineligible. If you like it and stay in, not only will you have wonderful experiences, but you'll have a very good pension and medical care all of your life." I said, "That's it." I came out of my shell. I got my driver's license when I was 26 years old. You didn't need to have a car in Chicago's mass transit system.

I went to Newport, Rhode Island, in October 1966. Prior to joining, I took two and a half months off to tour Europe on my own. I was ready to settle down with the Navy when I got to Newport. They made me lieutenant junior grade because I had the degree and several years of nursing experience.

My first hospital was Philadelphia. Shortly after my arrival, I said something stupid to a young Marine Corps officer with relatively minor injuries, but enough to send him home. It was something like, "Isn't it great that you will be going home?" He informed me, in no uncertain terms, that he had let his men, himself *and* the Marine Corps down by having to leave Vietnam. I learned an important lesson that day.

I had some psychiatric nursing experience. That's where I worked in Philadelphia. I found out that Navy nurses were not sent to Vietnam "en masse." Most of them were recommended by a supervisor. They assigned you to Vietnam if you had a critical skill like operating room or ICU, or you volunteered. I made it known I wanted to go. I got orders to Vietnam. I was not frightened because I had met patients who were back from Vietnam. I heard their stories and felt the camaraderie. I said it was time for me to go. My clinical supervisor saw to it that I got to go. I went to Vietnam in February 1968.

I was aboard the USS *Sanctuary*, AH17. My chief nurse was actually a nurse anesthetist. She would help in the OR suite. We worked very hard, six days a week and, often, more than an eight-hour shift. I knew nothing about Navy politics until a couple of years later. We just worked hard and well together and didn't "sweat the small stuff." I was a new lieutenant when I arrived aboard the hospital ship. My stripes, as full lieutenant, were waiting for me when I arrived. I didn't even know I had been selected. Mainly I was just a young kid working hard and looking for travel opportunities.

The first three months aboard USS *Sanctuary*, nurses were not allowed to leave the ship for anything. The commanding officer of the hospital was very protective of us and TET '68 was particularly busy. When the new CO arrived, we were allowed to go into Da Nang on a day off, two at a time, only when escorted by our Army liaison and MSC officer. Of course, it was to visit only military establishments. We were not allowed to "roam the street" going to Vietnamese restaurants or shops. As time progressed, we were allowed to accept organized group invitations from military land units for dinner parties and/or tours of their facilities. We were always treated like queens.

I worked mostly med-surg. Malaria was prevalent, as were flareups with peptic ulcers. Troops were to take an antimalaria pill weekly, which often made them sick with diarrhea. Some chose not to take it. We had a few deaths from malaria. The Falciparum strain seemed more difficult to treat than the Vivax. Within two weeks or so, most were back to duty. For ulcers, rest and regular meals had them back to duty in a few days. There was a death due to typhoid, which was particularly devastating for such a medical condition to be so lethal. Medical deaths were a bit harder to take for some of us.

There was really not a nurse in psychiatry, but I was the one who made rounds there and put out any minor fires. I found the Navy corpsmen well educated, especially if they had gone to a C school for psychiatric technician. It was a very small unit and the corpsmen ran it with the psychiatrist. They had anywhere from 10 to a maximum 20 patients at one time. Those diagnosed with situational reaction were ready to go back to duty rather quickly. If psychotic, it was believed that even if he had stayed home, the patient was prone to break down sooner or later.

We all took turns being in the recovery room. The recovery room was also pre-op. Each of us had a regular shift. About once a week you had an additional shift down in this pre-op area. We wore our nurse's white caps and our regular nurse's uniform. The patients would come to us, a majority of the time, by helicopter. They would arrive stripped of clothing and weapons, having had some morphine and IVs started. When they got to us, we monitored their care. The nurses aboard the USS *Sanctuary* had nothing to do with triage. Triage was a very small area. There were doctors, corpsmen, lab techs and a Chaplain there. Patients were not worried about their own wounds. They were worried about each other.

Aboard the other hospital ship, the USS *Repose*, they had an ICU nurse helping with the triage. Doing triage, you had to have your lab tech there to do the type and cross-matching. They had a chaplain, two or three doctors, and several corpsmen for moving patients, taking specimens or getting results. I'm glad we were spared triage because that was a very traumatic area. Sometimes the guys would die there before they had a chance to be treated. I remember the ones who were what they called "expectant." They were brought up to post-op, moved to the side, and a curtain drawn around them. I can still vividly picture a big, strong, strapping African American Marine with "Unknown American" written across his chest in black marker pen. He was still breathing, but there was really nothing they could do for him. All we did was watch him and hold his hand. He was beyond repairing, but still alive, in the technical sense. There were some guys who came without dog tags. At that time, I don't know what they did to identify him. I always wondered if this man had been MIA or were they somehow able to find out who he was.

We had a standard protocol once it was determined the patient was going to have surgery. They used a lot of Decadron, a cortico-steroid, and penicillin. We drew many labs. Everyone got the same thing unless they were allergic. We cared for Vietnamese enemies and civilians. We also cared for the Montagnards, the native Indian-like people who helped us during the war. I remember one lady was on a gurney with some kind of wounds and kept saying, "mundi, mundi." I didn't know what in the world she was talking about. She finally raised the sheet and pointed to her butt. She had to pee. Sign language is wonderful.

They were brave young men, 18 years old, and here they were being asked to do things beyond their level of maturity. That's one thing for the Marine Corps. They just instill in those young men qualities they would never get until they were much older, if ever. That's the overall feeling I saw and heard.

There was some levity when the Army was doing a lot of fighting. We would get a massive influx of Army patients. The few Marines we had around, at the time, would say, "Those Army guys don't know how to fight. Look at all of them in here." If the Marine Corps had been fighting, the Army guys would say the same thing about them. They would have the privilege of making a lighter situation out of something horrible.

They stayed with us as long as two weeks, then went back to duty or were medevacked for further treatment. Because of the animosity about the war, I thought some of these guys wouldn't want to go back to the rice paddies. On evacuation day, back to duty, I never ever saw anybody talk about not going back to their unit. They wanted to go back to their unit, Army and Marine Corps alike. They would sit around reading comic books until the helicopter came to take them back to their unit. Here we have the contrast of these men doing such manly things, but reading comic books, matching how young they really were.

Normally, the ship would go to the Philippines or someplace for maintenance every 90 days. By the time I got there in early February

1968, it was the hottest year of the war, very heavy casualties the whole year. We didn't go anywhere else because there was not enough time for the ship to be offline that long. We were on line 90 days or more at a time. Then we would go to the Philippines for four or five days. They would patch up the ship the best they could. We would go right back to work afterwards.

In the Philippines, we offloaded as many patients as we could, so we wouldn't have as many patients to take care of while we were doing R&R. There was a nice officers' club and we had a lot of fun buying things. We saved money but spent some of it on reel-to-reel tape record-ers, other electronic equipment, dishes, and other kinds of stuff. We were paid in cash. We each had a little locker on our desk, a metal safe. It had a code so we could keep valuables locked up in there. Two of us shared a room with metal bunk beds. I saved a lot of money, at least two-thirds minimum of every paycheck. We also received $60 a month, combat pay, because we were in a combat zone. There really weren't that many places to spend it. We didn't buy the big stuff until we were ready to go home. Then, we shipped it just like a regular PCS move. They came and packed us out. It was put on a barge and taken to some inland area where they did the actual Navy shipping procedure. I always received all of my belongings without any trouble. Coming out, I shipped a foot-locker with civilian clothes and extra uniforms. We carried a lot of our uniforms with us in suitcases for the actual arrival in Vietnam. Some-body had broken into my footlocker and took only a couple pairs of paja-mas and a blouse. Everything else was in there.

We had a Cambodian patient, who was a mercenary. They were in the war, too. He had TB. He had been in isolation in our medical ward. He was also a little bit delirious. I don't know if it was from drugs or what. One night he came, like a frightened rabbit, running through the nurses' quarters. We had to call security to subdue him.

There was the time when one of the nurses in a three-person room had a metal door bumper guard on an outside wall. Somehow some sail-ors had unscrewed that bumper guard, leaving a hole. This hole allowed a peep-hole. One of the girls, one evening, just happened to look over there and saw this eyeball. We had a peeping-tom from our own crew. I don't know if they found him, but believe me, that hole in the bulkhead was patched up very soon.

We were anywhere from five to ten miles offshore when fighting was limited. We cruised from Da Nang and points south, as far south as Chu Lai, all the way up to the DMZ. That was our cruising zone. We'd parallel any action that was on land. When we were close enough to shore, sometimes we'd get these beautiful little tropical birds. They would try to roost on the ship. Then of course, we'd dump trash. The bigger birds would dive after the trash. One day, a corpsman had captured one of these bigger birds. He quickly opened the nurses' quarters and threw this bird in. That was kind of funny.

I never worked so hard in my life, but I was never happier, professionally and personally. In my younger years, I was so naive it was much easier. It wasn't until much later that I started to become more critical of myself and other people. With most people, it goes in reverse. They get mellower when they get older. I didn't start speaking up for myself until I was well into my thirties. I saw what it was all about and decided I needed to be a little more assertive. Everything was a good learning experience. Now, if anything, I'm accused of talking too much. Before, I never had anything to say because I might be wrong. I thought I might make a fool of myself.

Near the end of my tour, while in the Philippines, some of our nurses complained to a group of supply ship officers that they missed taking a tub bath. Shortly thereafter, a blue bathtub was high-lined over to us during a replenishment at sea! After much "to do," two of our three shower stalls on the upper deck of the nurses' quarters were removed to make room for the tub. A promise was made to fill it sparingly. In the end, it was used only once, if at all.

When I was getting ready to leave the ship in late January 1969, I arranged for circuitous travel. A nurse friend and I were able to spend a couple of weeks in mainland Japan. We planned this trip ahead of time. They were not granting this privilege to everyone. We were very fortunate. We got it because the timing was right. Since we were not going to exotic ports for repair aboard the ship, like they had the year prior to my arrival, they allowed us to have the bonafide R&R experience, like the troops. I signed up for Bangkok. You got five free days that were not counted as leave time, and you could fly. Bangkok was very popular. It was close and it was rarely cancelled. Sometimes, R&R trips were cancelled because of a number of different things, such as a high patient count or lack of proper air transport. Australia, where I really wanted to go, was cancelled too many times. I thought I'd better take what I could when it was available. I was the only one from my hospital ship at the time to go. I ran into an Army nurse on the same airplane to Bangkok. We arranged to share a room to save money. She went her way. I went my way.

I had never been to the Orient. They fly you over with other R&R recipients on an American military plane. When you get to Bangkok, they talk to you about the country, what you should expect, what you should and shouldn't do. They had the few of us ladies leave the room.

Then, they talked to the young men alone, the usual pep talk about VD. One of the things that make me chuckle about that is they had a very strong talk about Thai girls being so shy. You must be proper with them. Once you leave the airport and got into town, those shy little Thai girls were obviously hooking. At least the guys had their education about being careful.

I took tours in the city and countryside. There are merchants all over the main river in small boats selling fresh meats. People in other little boats would buy the meat. There were flies all over the meat. That seemed to be the main mode of shopping for meat.

When it was time to leave the ship, I'd had enough death and dying. I was ready to leave the Navy. I was barely out for a year when I realized I had made a big mistake. I elected to work for a civilian hospital in the Chicago area. I wanted to work pediatrics because I liked young people. I was tired of everybody dying. I was put to work, and I didn't say no because I was a quiet and respectful girl, on a pediatric oncology ward. It was a lot more depressing than any war was. After about six or eight months of working there, instead of asking for a transfer, I just wanted to go back into the Navy. Fortunately, I was welcomed with open arms. They gave me the same orders from a year prior, which were to go to Hospital Corps School, Great Lakes, Illinois.

I truly enjoyed Hospital Corps School. I taught pharmacology and basic nursing skills to corpsmen. There was still the draft. We had as many as 75 new corpsmen starting every week. The maximum time in corps school was close to three months. Somewhere along the line, they changed it to 18 weeks. We had curriculum that would accommodate any length of time.

We had a program for college graduates that chose to go to corps school instead of becoming an officer. Some of those guys were just marvelous. They became the educational petty officers or they were in an accelerated program. We would coach them in such a way that they would finish the whole course much sooner. They were a unique group. Through this program you didn't have to do four years. If you came in through OCS it was an immediate four-year commitment. Nurses only had a two-year commitment at the time.

At corps school, we had nothing to do with choosing men for Vietnam. In Philadelphia we did. It was the supervisor's job to send names of who was being sent to Fleet Marine Force (FMF) School. Fortunately, it was easy most of the time. Our striker corpsmen, the corpsmen that were not psych techs yet, were particularly vulnerable to being sent to FMF School. More often than not, there were men within that group who wanted to go. So, that decision was a "piece of cake." It became particularly tough when we needed a quota and there was nobody in the categories I just mentioned. The choice was left up to our supervisor, with some input from the staff nurses. This was not a comfortable thing to do, as they might not come home alive if sent to Vietnam.

I remember one time I knew of a corpsman who was a psych tech and did very good work. He was eager to go because his dad had been in Korea prior. Unfortunately, he was the only one that got killed over there in just a matter of months. When I meet a corpsman here in San Diego, who has been to Vietnam, the first thing I say is "God bless you." The typical thing here in San Diego, if you run into any Vietnam vet, we say "welcome home" to each other. The Vietnam veterans weren't welcomed home at the end of the war. Now we are all welcoming each other home. The first time that was said to me, I said, "You're right. Thank you so much and the same to you."

I didn't particularly feel any bad vibes when I came home. I remember one time a civilian friend of mine was traveling with me while I was in uniform. She said, "Did you see the way those people were looking at you?" I said, "What?" I have had people claim we were given dirty looks, but I just ignored it, didn't see it or it didn't register, but I understand it happened. I was never spat upon or anything like that. I'll never forget telling this one guy I was hitting it off with that I had just gotten back from Vietnam. He said, "You're kidding! Not you!" He said it like it was really something bad to admit it, let alone be in the military. When I told male relatives, men in general, that had never been in the military themselves, I was going to join the Navy Nurse Corps, they said, "Only prostitutes and lesbians join the military." That is not true. At first, I would just get a little flustered. Later I told them, "We are there to do a job, just like any Jane Doe at any hospital anywhere. Civilian nurses do not enjoy the same camaraderie and benefits." That was an example of my getting stronger, by the way. It shut them up in a hurry.

After three years at Great Lakes, I got recruiting duty. I was living in Dallas, Texas, and was covering Oklahoma, Arkansas, northern Louisiana, and southeast Texas. I enjoyed going to different schools of nursing to give talks and to nursing conventions. By that time, 1973 to 1976, the Vietnam War was getting a more positive response and there were nothing but good wishes. Some people recognized my Vietnam service ribbons. People were much more grateful and understanding in general.

I was then chosen for graduate school. I had taken a course at Texas Women's University in Dallas in conjunction with Parkland Hospital. Because I had a couple of graduate credits, the Navy allowed me to stay there in Dallas and finish my master's at Texas Women's University in medical/surgical nursing with an educational focus. This is another example of baccalaureate nurses who came from the "old school." It had been about twelve years since I got my bachelor's degree. I think they had a hard time deciding what we needed to know. Of course, student and faculty backgrounds are always so varied. I had not had any physical assessment, per se. Very few baccalaureate schools were actually teaching it. I had to make up for that. I found it very difficult and very stressful because the Navy was paying for it and giving me my salary. I had to do it well. I did okay but being behind the eight-ball was extra trying. I wasn't the only one who found it that way, but I was the only military nurse there at the time. Nurses tend to form a close knit group. Those of us that were having trouble would coach each other and it worked out. I graduated in 1977. It took a full year. Fortunately, I didn't have to write a thesis. You could do the thesis route, but that would take much longer. Texas Women's University had a professional paper option. It's like a watered-down thesis. That is the route I chose. It's a good thing because otherwise it would have taken much longer to graduate.

Upon completion of my degree, I went to Camp Pendleton. I hadn't had ward duty for some time. However, I was thrown in to being the charge nurse on a very busy medical ward. I had a little trouble catching up. They didn't like to send people from recruiting duty to graduate school because there would be too many years off the beaten path. Having had corps school prior to that meant I had not been on the wards even longer. But I managed. It was hard catching up to the pace and new developments. By that time, I was selected for commander. I was on that busy medical ward for about a year. Then, I went to nursing education and finished up the three years at Pendleton.

From Pendleton I went to Okinawa for 18 months. They needed a chief of nursing education. It was quite the challenge. In Okinawa, the biggest thrust was to get everybody certified in basic life support. We did not do advanced cardiac life support. That was just in its early stages of development. We knew it was coming. We didn't have the instructors to do it over there. They were doing advanced cardiac life support training at Pendleton before I left. I never qualified for anything beyond basic life support instructor trainer.

I came back to San Diego for my last five years before retirement. I enjoyed teaching diabetics, which was one of my strengths. They allowed me to be in charge of diabetes education. I had my own patients to teach and went to the wards to relieve the nurses from the time it takes to teach people basic insulin administration skills. It is a job that any sharp lieutenant could have done. Fortunately, even as a commander, I think they were okay with me being in that job as a twilight tour. They knew it was getting done and getting done well.

I retired at the end of October 1987. Having been at Pendleton, I knew the area and I wanted to stay in southern California. I bought my first house in 1982. It is my last house. I'm sure I'll stay here forever. I am forever grateful having been a Navy nurse.

Elaine reflected further, at the time of this book's publication. "At 83 years of age, I am again asked to reminisce about the impact the Vietnam experiences had upon my life. These relatively new emotions I am experiencing, no doubt, stem from the fact that I feel that I may be experiencing some PTSD. Within the last three years, maybe fired by the relative isolation due to Covid and losing two significant people in my life, I am having more memories of Vietnam. A very recent trigger was during a chat with a person from the Philippines. As I spoke of fun times in that country that had been a respite from duty, I began to cry and had to stop the conversation. Typically, I do not have a depressive personality. However, I am plagued much more often now with unexpected emotions, specifically those feelings and memories related to Vietnam."

Ellen Komarek Duvall

I GRADUATED FROM Morton East High School in Cicero, Illinois, then from the University of Minnesota with a BSN. During my junior year, they talked to us about several different avenues of nursing. Military people were presenters, and that intrigued me. This was during the Vietnam era. The Air Force did not offer a financial incentive. I contacted both the Army and the Navy recruiters because they both had financial aid for nursing students.

I did pray about it, and decided I would join the service that contacted me within one week. I lived in a dorm and my mailbox was on the top row. I didn't think much about it but, sure enough, on Saturday, I received a letter from the Navy recruiter. It was three months before I heard from the Army. The Army recruiter phoned and said, "Well, it's time we get you in here for your physical." I said, "I've already joined the Navy."

The Navy paid for my senior year of college, including mandatory summer school, part of the nursing program back then. As soon as I graduated, I went to OCS (Officer Candidate School) in Newport, Rhode Island. I was there four and a half weeks in June. I received orders to Philadelphia Naval Hospital. I met three girls at OCS that were also going to Philadelphia and we got an apartment there together.

I started in psych, which was in the ramp area. Extending from the multistory hospital were two ramps (long wooden passageways) to ten wards. One ramp went to the ten orthopedic wards. Of the ten wards on the psych ramp, eight were psychiatric, one a neuro-geriatric. I worked the "seizure" ward (seizures and quadriplegic). Once, I got tangled in a circle-electric bed curtain. It ripped off my nursing cap. Of course, you have to be in uniform correctly. When I left the patient, I went to the corpsmen's desk. Using the glass door of the medicine cabinet as a mirror, I put my cap back on. After it was secured, with all bobby pins out of sight, I turned around and had four patients standing there watching me. They said, "We wondered how you gals kept those things on your head." That just cracked me up.

Many of the neuro-psych patients with seizures were up and about. I would also cover the ward. It was really like a nursing home with male veterans. At nighttime, we did rounds on all ten wards including the three locked wards. When patients first arrived, they were in a locked ward until they could be assessed. Then, they were transferred to one of the four wards until discharge. Some of the patients had character disorders, such as those who were sociopaths. The Navy would administratively discharge these. Several of the patients had significant problems. Of course, PTSD was not identified back then.

The patients earned "privileges" to go out into the community by doing assigned hospital jobs. Most of our patients did the cleaning because they were up and about, as opposed to the medical patients in the main building. Some would be patients on the wards where they were working. There was a lot of camaraderie between these patients. Our patients were Marines. Occasionally, we would have a sailor.

I got to Philly in August 1967. In December 1968, I detached and had all of 1969 on board the USS *Sanctuary*, completely staffed by Navy personnel. Today, our hospital ships are USNS = United States Navy Ship, staffed by Merchant Marines. The ship's crew is civilian and the hospital crew is Navy. I arrived the third week in January and was sent home the second week in December. I was fortunate that I had both Christmases at home. By then, they were winding the war down. Nobody knew it back home, but we knew it because that was the year, midway through 1969, they started pulling the Marines back. The Army was doing more of the forward and holding deployment processes supposedly in preparation for withdrawal. So, come the

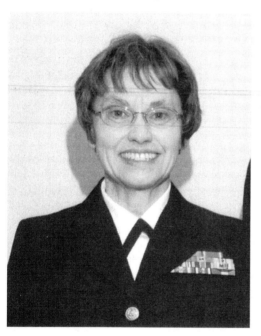

Ellen Komarek Duvall negotiated the ramps of naval hospitals, the narrow passageways of naval hospital ships and the desert military sites of Operation Desert Storm during her career as a U.S. Navy Nurse Corps officer. Photo by permission.

late summer and early fall, we noticed a significant drop in census. The hospital ships started coming home the next year. Veterans I meet now, if they served after 1972, are likely Army, not Marines.

I had become ill the night before I left the States for Vietnam. I was in the BOQ at Travis AFB and had eaten a nice dinner at the officers' club. That night, about 2:00 a.m., I awoke with vomiting and diarrhea. I thought, "Oh my gosh, I've got to check out at 11:00 and board a plane!" By 11:00 a.m., I had stopped vomiting, but was exhausted and felt terrible. I went to the airport, although the plane wasn't scheduled to leave until 10:00 p.m. I had no energy to do any sightseeing before heading to the airport. I was so drained I had no trouble sleeping on the plane. There were only three females among the passengers. The other two women were really envious that I could sleep. Today, I can't sleep on an airplane. We landed in Hawaii and Guam for refueling. They did allow us to get off the plane and walk around a little. I remember the heat. Each stop was hotter than the previous stop. When we got to Da Nang, the heat was stifling.

All three of us were going to the *Sanctuary*. One was a lieutenant commander, thus senior to us two JGs. We thought she knew Navy protocol related to boarding a ship. She said, "I've never been to a ship. I don't know any more than you." None of us had ever been overseas. We stood out because we were the only ones in blue and white pinstripe uniforms. Everyone else was in green Marine cammies and Army battle dress.

A nurse that I knew on the ship, now living in Canada, was diagnosed with PTSD fifteen years after she got back. She worked with the children aboard the ship. She kept having nightmares about these little ones. She left nursing but went into chaplaincy. As a chaplain in a hospital, she worked with people who were dying, which is probably the worst thing she could have done. Somehow, she got to D.C. for the dedication of the Women's Vietnam Memorial. She talked with other vets who surmised that she had PTSD and insisted that she get into counseling. She went into counseling at the VA for about three months. She now has her doctorate. She left working as a chaplain in a hospital and is teaching theology in a Catholic seminary. To me, Vietnam was just another year of my life and I was not traumatized.

We landed in Da Nang and the ship was not there. Ordinarily the ships cruised between Da Nang and the DMZ. I think it is about a forty- or fifty-mile area. It turned out our XO was on the same plane we were on as he boarded in Hawaii after R&R. The XO was a plastic surgeon who often repaired cleft palates on the children. Knowing more *Sanctuary* nurses were expected, he introduced himself to us in Da Nang and said, "Stay with me." We tagged along as he breezed through the airport and went to a small office and said, "What did you do with my ship?" When we flew over the harbor in Da Nang, he saw that the ship wasn't where it was supposed to be. Apparently there had been an offensive (a "push") south of Da Nang. Ordinarily the hospital ships didn't go any further south than Da Nang. We would need to "chopper down" to board the ship in Cam Ranh Bay.

First, we spent a night in quarters of the Navy tent hospital in Da Nang to await transportation to the ship. I got to visit one of my corpsmen that had been injured and was a patient there. That night we got to bed at 7:00 p.m. and slept like logs. Apparently, there was an air raid during the night. When the alarms go off you are supposed to either go to a bunker or get under the bunk beds. There were two half-inch-thick foam mattresses and flak jackets under our bunks. We were supposed to put on a flak jacket and get under the bottom bunk. None of the three of us even heard the sirens.

We had to helicopter down to our ship in what they called Grasshoppers, which were Air Force helicopters. They weren't like the helicopters that the Marines used. These helicopters were double deck in height. It was my first helicopter ride. There might have been a dozen enlisted men who were also coming back from R&R and returning to the ship, so we went in two helicopters. I looked forward to seeing a nurse that I had known in Philadelphia who was from my hometown on the ship. She had been ordered to the *Sanctuary* a year before I was. Our two tours should have overlapped. However, my arrival got pushed ahead from December to the end of January. Her departure from the ship was moved back from February to January. She boarded the first helicopter in our party. I was on the second, circling overhead. I never even got to see her or give her a hug.

There were two of us to a room in the nurses' quarters. I had a top bunk. In those days, I was young and could climb up there without any trouble. Every drawer and locker had a latch on it of course, so when the ship rolled, they wouldn't open. There was a sink in the room with a bowl that was only about a foot across. Down the hall/passageway was where the toilets and showers were. We had to take the classic Navy shower where you turn the water on, get wet, turned the water off, wash, then you turn the water on and rinse. All the water had to be filtered and desalinated. They were very restrictive on how much water we could use because filtered water had to be used for cooking, laundry, etc. Toilet water was saltwater. Every three months, the ship would go into port in Subic Bay, Philippines, for cleaning and maintenance work. Saltwater is hard on ships. In fact, apparently the ship had been scheduled to go into Subic, but it was held "on station" because of the push south of Da Nang. The ship had been "on-line" for 120 days instead of the customary 90. There was a big crowd when the ship finally did get to Subic because we were online for so much longer than even the "gray Navy" ships. I found that Navy ships are in port more than I ever realized. Regular sailors considered the 90 days that hospital ships are normally at sea to be long, thus being on-line more than 100 days was deserving of a celebration. It was also a hospital ship record. I came aboard at the tail end of the 100-plus days. The second-year crew was really ready to get off the ship once we reached Subic.

When I came aboard the *Sanctuary*, I was at the very beginning of the third crew. People rotated in and out over about a six or eight-week span. I was assigned to the medical ward. The medical wards were primarily filled with malaria patients. They had one huge ward that had 102 beds. One half of the ward was smaller with two-tiered bunks, called racks in Navy lingo. The other half part was larger in deck space, and bunks were three high. Malaria patients were kept until they completed their medications, then returned to duty.

There are five different kinds of malaria and there were two in Vietnam. Each is treated differently. One was Falciparum malaria and the second, Vivax, was sensitive to Chloroquine. The Falcip patients had to be on medication three weeks. The other, only 10 days. We had to keep them on board ship until they could return to full duty. Because we needed their racks for our sicker people, once stabilized, they would be transferred to the "medical holding ward" down in the hold of the ship. No portholes there and all the bunks were three tiered. These patients would have one corpsman for the whole 100 or so patients to monitor for relapses until they could return to full duty in the war zone.

On the medical ward, we had a microscope and made blood slides. The ward physician diagnosed which malaria the Marine had. Bypassing the lab meant we could get them on meds faster. Many of the doctors were lieutenants, probably pretty fresh out of medical school and internship. I do remember we had one patient that had ulcerative colitis, not dysentery. When I saw him, it reminded me of the death camps of Nazi Germany. He was so emaciated. He arrived walking, but his thinness and his hollowed eyes showed he was starving. I wondered if he survived. Ward officers wanted him medevacked ASAP. He would die, as we didn't have the treatment needed to meet his nutritional demands.

Another medical concern would be dysentery. I came on duty one morning and the corpsman's desk was covered with stool specimens. The patients had come in with diarrhea. A usual order was to obtain three stool specimens from the patient to identify what organism was causing the diarrhea. However, many were dragging their heels turning in their specimens. We weren't able to diagnose them, and they could stay aboard longer. The corpsman told them that if they didn't give him some specimens by morning, the nurse was going to give them enemas. Thus, that morning he got his specimens. There was no way I would have done that, but the patients didn't know that.

A Deck was medical, B Deck was the Vietnamese women and children's ward, orthopedic and urology wards. If surgical patients weren't able to return to full duty in five days, we would medevac them, primarily to Japan. There were three wards on B and two wards on A Deck. The SOQ, sick officers' quarters, actually had patient rooms with two bunks per room. On C Deck there were three wards, two surgical wards and an ICU. The bunks aboard the ships were anchored down. They are called racks for a reason. It is like a big shelf with one-inch diameter pipe all the way around it, instead of side rails. The mattress was about four inches thick. The upper and lower bunks were anchored on their sides to poles at the head and the foot. When they weren't in use, they could actually be hinged up to a 60-degree angle. Then, they could be lowered again to a 90-degree angle, parallel to the floor. They were held in that position by a strip of metal, maybe two inches wide, that came down like a big hook. One length of the bunks was attached to the poles and the outside of the upper bunk was hooked to the overhead (ceiling) at the head and foot. The lower bunk outside was hooked to the upper bunk.

The ICU beds were beds, not racks, and were on wheels. On the *Repose*, the other hospital ship in Vietnam, the beds did not have wheels. We could move our beds within the ICU ward. There were maybe a dozen beds in ICU. They had to be kept tied to poles so they wouldn't move.

I was never assigned in ICU when I worked on B Deck. I did go there a couple of times to mix IVs for those patients. In those days we, not the pharmacy, mixed our own IVs. We usually put vitamins in them or penicillin. We combined penicillin and sulfa in the same IV bottle, no plastic bags in 1969, which I learned a few years later, wasn't a good idea. We didn't know that then. Cephalosporins, like today's Keflex, were just beginning to come in. Those were piggybacked to the main IV. There was something that we piggybacked that was sticky. It may have been penicillin. One of the surgical wards that I did work occasionally was primarily abdominal surgeries. The other ward was thoracic. We had chest tubes and Gomcos, suction for nasogastric tubes. Both of those had glass bottles. Whenever they were to be used, they had to be secured. Chest bottles were taped to the deck. One leg of the Gomco would be anchored to one of the poles so it wouldn't roll. Whenever there were rough seas of any degree, we would tape the IV bottles to their metal poles so they wouldn't sway, risking breakage.

The ship was always on a gentle roll, so everything in quarters, as well as the wards, was to be secured. We had an ensign line officer piloting the ship coming back into harbor in Da Nang one morning and the ship took a big roll. Anything that people didn't have anchored fell. I know a couple of gals were furious because they had speakers on their stereo systems and they went flying. Personal items were not secured. We had become complacent, since the seas were relatively smooth.

I remember the physician in the abdominal ward saying that he would not give patients sleeping pills. Of course, they knew nothing about PTSD in those days. He said, "When he's tired enough, he'll sleep. We don't want to get him on sleeping pills." In Vietnam, marijuana and drug trafficking was a major concern.

We had Vietnamese patients. We did have two Vietnamese interpreters. The U.S. military arrested one of them because he was supplying some of our people with drugs. The marijuana in Vietnam was stronger than what was in the States. I remember walking through one of the decks and seeing this young man just sitting there waiting to be taken off ship. Once he was gone, we didn't know what happened to him. The interpreters we had were in the South Vietnamese Army and they would be the ones disciplining him. Several corpsmen voiced concern that with the U.S. wanting him off the ship, it would be interpreted as "losing face" in their culture and might cost him his life.

On C Deck, going down the passageway from the surgical wards, was C4, a psych ward. One evening when the ward officer and I were at supper, one of the patients on C4 had a seizure. Unable to contact us, the corpsman called the officer of the deck, to get help. When I got there, they were taking the patient up to the medical ward. The OOD commended the corpsman for his quick problem solving.

The ship would go into Subic Bay every three months. We tried to cut down our census. They would be admitted to the *Repose* or Da Nang Naval Hospital. Our highest census was 412. Supposedly the ships could carry about 350. One reason we wanted to offload most of our patients before we went to Subic was that the ship was in for repairs and many areas of the ship, especially in the patient areas, would be without air conditioning. The ventilation would be off. It's like working in a metal box, so air needed to be piped in. If you don't have that, what you have is like a small gymnasium after a wrestling match, hot and sticky.

One night when I was on duty and in Subic, we had three or four wards with patients. I was making rounds and only one of my wards had cool air. The patients were pretty sticky and hot, as well as the staff. In one ward, there was a young man who was spiking a temperature to 104 degrees. The corpsman called his buddy, who was corpsman in one of the other wards. It did have air conditioning. He had an empty bed. He asked me if he could move this guy into this other ward. I didn't know if I had the authority to do that, but I told him to go ahead and move him. He was ambulatory. We bundled him up and walked him down to the other ward. He was a young Marine and felt like hell, but he just got up and started walking. In a civilian hospital, a wheelchair would have been needed.

I do remember a couple of times, when fighting was slack, we somehow kept getting patients with fractured jaws. It seemed that Marines, if they weren't fighting the enemy, they were fighting each other. I can remember a couple of them with their wired jaws "eating" via a straw.

Midway through, in June 1969, Army Lieutenant Sharon Lane was killed by shrapnel. Her hospital received a direct hit. Of the eight nurses on The Wall, she is the only one killed by enemy fire. I wonder if it happened on the day I remember we had mass casualties, like we never had before. In Vietnam, the money that was used was called scrip. We did not use U.S. bills because of the risk for counterfeiting. Periodically, they would change the color of the bills to undercut black marketing. That money was supposed to be used on American instillations only. It was not supposed to be in the Vietnamese economy. If you were buying or selling anything in the Vietnamese economy, you were to use Vietnamese piasters. However, the black market didn't adhere to that. In past times, when they would do this exchange, they would give advance notice to make sure our military personnel had all their scrip on the day of the exchange. What was happening was that GIs, who were dealing in the black market, would get their Vietnamese buddies to give back all their scrip. The GI would get it exchanged, and reimburse their Vietnamese buddy.

In mid–1969, they did the exchange but gave no one advance notice. The morning came and bases were locked down. The Vietnamese were not allowed on base while the money was exchanged. The Vietnamese couldn't get the scrip they had received back to the GIs when this exchange occurred. Anybody that had the old scrip, by 5:00 p.m. that night it was totally worthless. Who knows how many hundreds of dollars were lost. The Vietnamese were furious. That night the Viet Cong really hit us. The Navy hospital in Da Nang was hit. I assume the hospital where Lt. Lane worked was also hit.

Da Nang Naval Hospital was deliberately hit. From a nearby mountain, the enemy lobbed in a rocket and it was short. The next landed closer and the third hit the hospital. Once they hit the hospital itself, they lobbed in several more. Meanwhile, the two hospital ships were in the midst of their rotation. One ship was always up north by the DMZ. She would cruise around up there for three days. The other hospital ship would be in Da Nang harbor. The ship that was in Da Nang would leave at 5 p.m. and cruise north, arriving at the DMZ about midnight. After reporting "on station," the other ship would cruise south and about 7 a.m. would enter Da Nang harbor and be there for two and a half days. Every three days the ships would rotate. Thus, every three nights, there would be no hospital ship in Da Nang. There was always a ship at the DMZ because there was no other U.S. hospital that far north.

The night Da Nang hospital was included in the assault, there was no hospital ship in the harbor. At 0700 when we reached the harbor, we still had not dropped anchor when helicopters were calling to land. I'm sure the command staff aboard ship knew what had happened, but the rest of us did not. The Da Nang hospital had all they could do to handle their own casualties. Thus, the wounded in the field waited all night for a hospital ship to arrive. We heard the call for corpsmen to report to the helicopter deck. A corpsman from every ward would report respond to be litter bearers. Two corpsmen would carry a stretcher to our small triage area and then to x-ray, pre-op prep, etc. The next thing we heard was "all off duty lab techs report to the lab. All off duty x-ray techs report to x-ray." That was our first warning that something big was occurring.

They just kept bringing in wounded Marines from the field. The ORs went until midnight that night. Helicopters did not fly to the ships after dark. I wonder if that night was the night that Sharon Lane was killed. She was at an Army hospital in Chu Lai on June 8, when it was hit. She was the only woman to be killed by hostile fire in Vietnam.

During the day, we had a nurse assigned to each ward. On evening shift one or two nurses would be assigned for the deck. That day, I was on C Deck working in the abdominal surgical ward and also helped mix IVs in ICU. By 5 p.m., the evening nurse had not come to get report from me. I went looking for her and found her on the thoracic surgical ward. In those days, patients with chest tubes were kept in ICU. There were eight patients with fresh chest tubes on that ward. I took one look at her and told her I would cover the other ward for the evening. There was no way she could cover the thoracic ward and the abdominal ward, too.

On the abdominal surgery ward, by evening we had about eight patients with nasogastric tubes to suction (i.e., fresh post-op abdominal surgeries). I think every Gomco on board ship was in use. About 2300 I was making a final walk through the ward in preparation for the night nurse, hoping I was going to get relieved. The patients had little lights if they wanted to read in their bunks. As I got to the back of the ward where it was pretty dark, we are talking 36 bunks, I was stopped by two or three different patients who were reading and had their lights on. They had picked out which of those guys were the sickest and most injured. They were going to try and stay awake during the night. One said to me, "Tell the doc (meaning the corpsman) I'll keep an eye on so-and-so. If he needs a urinal or anything, I'll get it for him." I have never run into that in civilian work before or since. These guys were Marines and all buddies and they knew who was severely injured. They knew the staff was swamped. I was so impressed with the way the patients stepped forward to help their buddies.

As night fell, the helicopters stopped coming and surgeries finally ended. The situation became manageable and the night nurse was able to cover both wards. I was relieved to get to my bunk after midnight.

Nobody in an upper bunk would have been on an IV, only the lower rack patients. The way you had to handle that was the antibiotics we gave went into Volutrols, the way you would for pediatric patients. There was a little cylinder. The nurse injected the medication in there, ran 100 ml of the main IV fluid into the chamber, put the antibiotic in the chamber, and that dripped down into the patient. When it emptied out, the main IV just refilled. We were doing the penicillin like that. That meant we could hang the IV bottle from the hook, stand on the deck, reach up to the upper bunk, and on that hook, you could hook your bottle. The problem was when you had a Volutrol, an IV device for giving up to 100 ml of fluids, that hung below the primary IV bottle. We had to lift the bottle on the highest hook on the bar holding the upper rack. The only way I could reach that high was to stand on the rail of the lower bunk. We would stand on the frame at the foot of the bed, because we were in skirts. In 1969, there were no pant uniforms for nurses. We would look around, hoping nobody was paying attention, and take a giant step up onto the rail. I'd have to wrap my left arm around that metal pole that was holding the rack and grab the bottle with my left hand. With my right hand, I could reach up to the top of the Volutrol and inject the medication.

I was in the middle of that very undignified pose, trying not to fall, when in walked one of our MSC (medical service officers). He was touring two Marine generals to present purple hearts. He took one look and gasped. He looked at me, looked at them and said, "That is one of our Navy nurses." I said, "I'm sorry, this is the only way I can do this." Fortunately, they saw the humor in it. We had to improvise with the equipment and circumstances we had. All this avoided giving intramuscular injections to our patients because of the risk of abscesses with the newer antibiotics. Those patients were getting a lot of antibiotics.

On B Deck, orthopedics, pseudomonas infection was common. There were many, too many, that came in with limbs blown off, a lot of traumatic amputees, because of land mines. The Vietcong would put any garbage they could into the land mine to inflict extensive damage and infection when it exploded. When the wounded came in, they were contaminated with pseudomonas. The B Deck reeked of pseudomonas. Even today I think if I smelled pseudomonas, I would know it.

We had met two lady missionaries that ran an orphanage in Da Nang. There were several mission orphanages. I had become friendly with our chaplain aboard ship. He had "adopted" this particular orphanage. Staff from the ship had gone there several times. When I was to rotate off the ship, I needed to stay in Da Nang a couple of days to await my flight to "the world" (the USA). My ship was going up north to the DMZ. I disembarked before it left Da Nang harbor. I received permission to spend those few days at the mission with the missionaries. I didn't want to just sit in the nurses' transit quarters within the nurses' area in Da Nang hospital. The mission had a Christmas program. I helped sort clothes and do other chores to help them. My time there seemed beneficial to them and to me.

When I flew home, I do not remember much about the flight. I might have been the only woman on board. I flew into Norton AFB, San Bernardino area. I remember when I got back, they had buses that were going to take us from the Air Force base to LAX. At Norton, I got out of my light blue uniform, threw it away, and put on my service dress blues, the winter uniform, as it was mid–December. I was flying back to Chicago. I didn't have my uniform coat, so that was all I had to keep me warm. By the time I changed and got out of the terminal to catch the bus to LAX with fellow Vietnam passengers, it must have been one of the last buses because it wasn't totally full. I do remember I was the only woman on the bus. As we rode to LAX, the guys kept their voices low because I'm sure they were well aware of my presence. One of the guys did blurt out, "Look at that girl. She has half a dress on. She forgot her dress." I was thinking the exact same thing. Before I went to Vietnam, girls wore what we called a car coat, which came several inches above the knees. Our dresses came just below our knees. The year before I had left home, hemlines really started shortening. Miniskirts were all the rage in 1969. When I got back in December 1969, girls were wearing skirts that came to their mid-thighs. This was one of the things that changed while I was gone. Who paid attention to fashion in Vietnam? Who cared? I remember when I had been aboard ship, a couple of the guys had gone for R&R down to Australia and commented that Navy nurses needed to be shortening their skirts. Our uniform skirts covered our knees, per regulation. Our skirts were now six inches too long, compared to the styles in Australia and certainly apparent on the streets of LAX.

The men with long hair created another rash of bus comments. When we were in Vietnam, short hair was regulation and desirable in the heat and dirt. When we got back to the States, the culture changes just hit us in our faces, the style, the clothing differences, and the hippie look we forgot about when we were over there. We returnees came from a country where people were starving and trying to figure out where they were going to get the next meal. In the States, people were trying to decide what size color television to buy. The difference in value structure hit me. How very different we are in all that we are blessed with. I would think of the poverty we saw in Vietnam and, of course, the tremendous destruction. I think it would be interesting to go back to see Vietnam now.

I was processed out of the Navy at Great Lakes. I had to stay in at least four more weeks to make sure I hadn't come down with any exotic diseases. I was released the first week of February 1970.

Eighteen years later I signed up with the reserve. It was a time of President Reagan and Oliver North. I was appalled that LCDR North would hide papers in his secretary's blouse and sneak them out the door to avoid authorities with warrants. He is not a hero to me.

At that time, I was on a flight and the man that was sitting next to me was an Army colonel. He asked me to join the Army, as they really needed nurses. I said, "If I ever join it would be the Navy, but I'm too old." He said people with previous service could get an age-waiver. By the end of the flight, he had me thinking.

I joined the reserve in time to be mobilized to Desert Storm, January 1991. We were Fleet Hospital Six in Bahrain. It is a country, not a city in Saudi Arabia, as some people thought. There was a 25-mile causeway between the island of Bahrain and Saudi Arabia. Like being on the *Sanctuary*, I felt it was a safe environment.

We were in Bahrain only two months, until the end of 1991. We got there about five days after the shooting war started. We were in tents on land owned by British Petroleum. The British expatriates set up our berthing tents and our bunks. Once we arrived, under the direction of the Seabees, we erected a 500-bed tent hospital in record time. Scuds did go overhead once or twice. My concern was if one was shot down over us, would the debris be hot? How flammable were the canvas tents we were in?

Reservists primarily staffed Fleet Marine Six and Fifteen. Active-duty personnel staffed the fleet hospital that had deployed in August

1990. We could walk out of our base during certain hours of the day and go to the ex-pat town. It had what they called a Cold Store where we could buy soda and snacks. There was a library there and we met some British ladies that worked there. Most were volunteers. They had a table display of books and information about the Middle East. They said, "Oh yes, we know where you're at because we helped put up the tents." That is how I learned the community worked with the Seabees. They were telling us how they were very concerned because they didn't like Saddam Hussein and were fearful for themselves. They were really pleased to have our installation there.

The U.S. government wanted to get reserve units out as soon as possible for several reasons. Reservists were expensive because we included numerous captains and senior enlisted. In addition, if they kept us beyond 90 days, we would be eligible for veteran benefits. Also, Ramadan was approaching. They had us back to the States before the end of March.

Fleet Hospital Six was basically a way station for medevac patients on their way to the airport and Germany. We were not busy and had only a handful of patients. The thing that I found interesting was the number of Vietnam veterans in the ranks. I remember one of the nurses saying that he was glad to come to this war because for once he'd like to come home a hero. Another person who had been enlisted during Vietnam was a commander now. Although he didn't go to Vietnam, his Stateside duty had been to accompany bodies to their families and attend the funerals of Vietnam dead. He was having flashbacks. He was now a psychologist and was one who was sent to talk with the U.S. POWs in treatment after release. One of our planes had crashed and the Iraqis held the crew. He said, "I saw in their faces some of the same looks I remember seeing in families back home during Vietnam." One of our corpsmen had been a Marine in Vietnam. He said, "I grew up in a small town and I wasn't a killer. When I came back people would cross the street so they wouldn't have to say hello to me. Some called me a baby killer. I never killed a baby. I'll never live in a small town again." When we were deployed, he was in the process of moving to Kansas City.

When I came home from Vietnam, people did not associate a woman, even when in uniform, with Vietnam. I did not endure negative harassment, as the men did. Today, as a woman vet, I also am not recognized for serving, although I served in two wars. When I occasionally attend a veteran related function, people will thank men and totally ignore me. I still remember the first time, 30-some years after my year in Vietnam, that a stranger said "thank you for your service" to me. I was in uniform in a restaurant, as it was our reserve drill weekend.

When I returned to the table, I sat stunned. I told my reserve friends that someone had just thanked me for my service. The others were nonchalant. I replied, "You don't understand. I'm a Vietnam vet and that is the first time anyone has ever thanked me for serving."

Since 9–11, servicemen are showered with "thank you for your service." Vietnam veterans have been able to ride those coattails to receive recognition that was lacking for decades. Yet, women vets continue to be on the periphery and discounted. I don't wear ball caps nor jackets plastered with military insignia. But women who do wear ball caps with "Woman Veteran" emblazoned, and pins saying "Woman Veteran," tell me they are ignored. Deep down I guess I continue to carry resentment for the shabby treatment Vietnam veterans endured then and for decades after 1975.

Anne Kuhn Gartner

I GRADUATED FROM Magnificat High School in Rocky River, Ohio, in 1964. When I was in high school, there weren't a lot of choices, especially in an all-girls school. You either were in the college, secretarial or homemaking prep. I'd always played nurse and I think it just kind of stuck. When I first decided to go into nursing, I looked at a number of nursing schools. Because my mother went to St. Vincent Charity Hospital School of Nursing, I decided that is where I wanted to go also.

My mother was an industrial nurse. She worked for Warner and Swasey in Cleveland, Ohio, most of her career. She went back to hospital nursing when my sister and I were in sixth and seventh grades, working in the emergency room at St. Vincent Charity Hospital. She finished her career in the late 1970s. She was well known at the hospital I attended. The one rotation I did not do in nursing school was the emergency room. I didn't want to work there because everyone would call me "Micky's daughter." We could take different options. I really liked surgery. So instead of doing the ER, I did the OR.

In 1967, I graduated from nursing school. Before I graduated, the school had different organizations come in and talk about different areas of nursing. It was at this time the military services came in. The woman that came from the Navy was a commander at the time. She was very instrumental in opening my eyes to military nursing. I looked at the Army and the Air Force, but decided the Navy really had more to offer. The uniform worked, too.

I was a senior at the time, so I filled out all the Navy's paperwork. My mother had to help me because she was born in Cuba. There were a lot of questions to answer. It took a little longer for my papers to be processed because, even though she was an American citizen (her father and mother were American), she was still born in Cuba. They had to do an investigation. I finally got a letter from the Navy right before I graduated in August.

After I finished nursing school, I was working as a graduate nurse

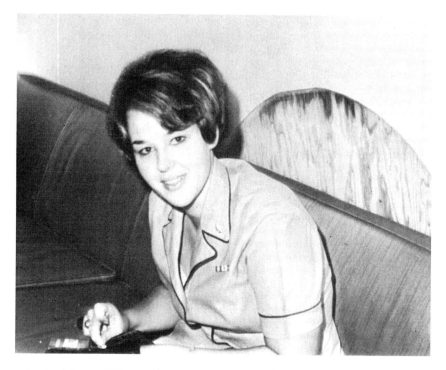

Captain Anne Kuhn Gartner in the nurses' lounge. Photo by permission.

at Lakewood Hospital in the PACU [Post Anesthesia Care Unit]. The reason I was working there is because a friend of my mother's, another nurse, was working there. She encouraged me to get critical care experience if I was going into the military. She convinced me to work in the PACU. I also needed to take my state boards. In Ohio, boards sat once a year. I worked as a graduate nurse, GN, until I took my boards in November. We went down as a class to take the boards. Because I was getting ready to go into the military, and needed to have my board results before I was commissioned, I sat in a separate section. Our tests were hand scored. There were about forty of us going into different military services. On November 20 I got my board results. My mother was at home. I was working. She called me on the phone and said, "You can now write 'RN' after your name."

I was commissioned November 30, 1967. I received the dates for OCS, Officer Candidate School, at Newport, Rhode Island. I was scheduled to report in on 31 December. In the interim, I scrambled to get all of the "stuff" I needed to take. When I first went into the military, they gave me a list of items I was supposed to take. A black cocktail dress and a nice purse they thought would be important because you were expected to attend various functions. You were expected to be properly dressed. I can remember going to Higby's Department Store in Cleveland and looking for the typical black cocktail dress. "I found it!"

OCS lasted six weeks. It was bitter cold there. I can remember getting all our uniforms. At the time, we had all the hoods and havelocks as part of our uniform. They don't give those uniform parts out anymore. The middle of February was our graduation from Newport. My mom and dad drove from Cleveland, Ohio, to Newport, Rhode Island. There was a horrible snowstorm the day we decided to start driving back. We got stuck somewhere in Pennsylvania and had to spend the night. It took us three days to get back home.

My first duty station was Naval Hospital Corpus Christi, Texas. I reported to Corpus Christi in early March. I stayed in the BOQ, Bachelor Officers Quarters, because I didn't have a car. I started out working in all of the different wards. The first place they put me was my least favorite part of nursing, the psych ward. After about a month, I pleaded to get out of this ward. They said, "We'll put you on the surgical ward" and I said, "I'll take anything else." We had to rotate through all the wards and all the shifts, nights and PMs. After a while, I thought there's got to be a better way to do this. It was 1968 when a number of hospital corpsmen and nurses headed off to Vietnam. We had two nurses that came off the USS *Repose.* They painted a picture of how wonderful nursing was aboard a ship.

I had a friend at Corpus Christi who took me under her wing. She was a lieutenant. We would be on the different schedules together. I worked ICU and she worked the surgical ward. She really taught me to be a Navy nurse. I learned how to understand my patients, especially the patients who were coming back from Vietnam. They had been through a lot. Their psyche was fragile. They had a lot of flashbacks of their time in Vietnam. I really wanted to make a difference in how I cared for them. My friend introduced me to the "dream sheet." She told me to go to the hospital administration section and fill it out with the hope of getting into an area I wanted. I decided I wanted to go to Vietnam and help care for the soldiers, sailors and Marines before they were sent back Stateside for further medical care.

I went to the administrative office and filled out my dream sheet. I went back the next month and the admin tech in the office said, "You know, it would be a lot easier if you would just sign a whole bunch of dream sheets. I'll send them in every month." One place that I put was Vietnam on a hospital ship. Also, my friend had been to Iceland and really loved it. So, I put Naval Station Hospital Iceland. I was in Corpus Christi about eight months.

Normally orders came through normal channels, not as speed orders or orders across the teletype. Someone was scheduled to be sent a certain place, but an illness or family emergency happened that precluded that person from being sent there. They needed to have a replacement as quickly as possible. One night I was working and a set of speed orders came in for me to report to Hospital Ship USS *Sanctuary* (TAH-17). I spent 30 days' leave at home in order to get ready. I was to report in early February 1969. In the interim, I visited my friend from Corpus Christi who was instrumental in my being a better Navy nurse. She was now at Georgetown going through the nurse anesthetist program. She really set me in the right direction and did a lot to make sure when I went to Vietnam, I was prepared for whatever came along.

I headed for Vietnam, flying from Ohio to Los Angeles, then San Bernardino Air Force Base. The contract airlines flew out of that base. It seemed like we were in the air flying forever. The first flight started out at 11:00 p.m. We landed in Hawaii, stayed for about an hour, took off to Guam, and finally, on to Vietnam, landing in Da Nang. It took about 28 hours. Every three or four hours they fed us. I was one of two or three women on the plane. At the time, very few women were going to Vietnam. Most who did were nurses. There were no female pilots. There were a few women who worked admin and some other women on the bigger bases, like Da Nang. On my plane, there were one or two other women, not nurses.

We arrived in Da Nang very early in the morning. The hospital ships steamed off the coast of Vietnam. There were two hospital ships, the USS *Sanctuary* and the USS *Repose*. I went to the *Sanctuary*. If the ship was not in port, you could hook a ride with a chopper that was going out to deliver mail. If they were in port, you would take a launch out to the ship. I was lucky because they said in two days there was a helicopter going out to the ship to deliver the mail. I had to stay in Da Nang at the station hospital there. I didn't have to work at the hospital, but they put you through this whole safety course. Da Nang was pretty active in terms of the war.

They put us into temporary quarters and gave us our flak jacket, helmet, and instructions if the sirens went off. However, after being on a plane for so many hours, all I really wanted to do was just die. I went to bed. You always kept your flak jacket and helmet next to your bed. In case something happened, you could put it on very quickly. A weird noise woke me up. Someone came running through, yelling to get our flak jackets and helmets on and get under our bunks. Back then we used to wear curlers in our hair. Have you ever tried to put a helmet on with curlers in your hair? I put the flak jacket on, put the helmet on as well as

I could, and crawled under the bed. They finally came and woke me up after it was all over. I was asleep because I was so tired.

The next day I was to fly out to the ship. At that time, we wore light seersucker uniforms, the perfect uniform for Vietnam. We still had to wear covers (hats), but you couldn't keep the regular cover on. We were also allowed to wear these triangle scarves tied under our chin to keep our cover from flying away. These scarves were part of the Red Cross uniform. You were only allowed to wear your scarf when you were trying to get on a helicopter. Once you were in the helicopter you could take it off. It was just one of the weird things we did because there just weren't that many women. They had to make sure we knew not to let these covers go flying off into the blades of the chopper. The guys just took their covers off, but because we were "ladies" we weren't allowed to go uncovered.

We flew out to the ship. I was sitting on mail bags. There were tons of mail because they only took the mail out every so often. We were flying in on a big, double rotor Sea Stallion helicopter. There were all these people on the flight deck. They were cheering. I thought, "They're so happy to see me." Actually, they were excited to get the mail. Mail was so important for the staff to keep them connected to family and home.

The nurse who was leaving, whom I was replacing, was very happy to see me, so she could go back home. Nurses could only stay a year. The corpsmen could opt for a second year. But nurses and physicians were only allowed one year. There were so many who wanted to come over, they limited the time. Most of the corpsmen were drafted. They didn't want to be there any longer. Some of them did because they could make more pay. If they did two tours, they were guaranteed a Stateside billet and not going back with the Marines.

I got oriented to the ship and did the same type of rotations: nights, PMs and days, which depended on your seniority. I started working on the international ward. We took care of quite a few of the Vietnamese children, especially the ones that had cleft palates and other facial reconstructive issues. We had a plastic surgeon who did quite a few surgeries on these children. Our international ward had all the major medical services. We performed surgery 24 hours a day, if need be. We did rotate through all the areas, including medical. We had a lot of patients brought in with malaria. I ended up working mostly in the surgical areas, such as urology and ENT. We also had nurses working down in PACU. Most of the time, you had to have a lot of seniority to work in PACU, so I didn't get to work there. The operating room was strictly for nurses that had been through the Navy OR school. They really did need OR nurses that were already fully trained in the operating room. We

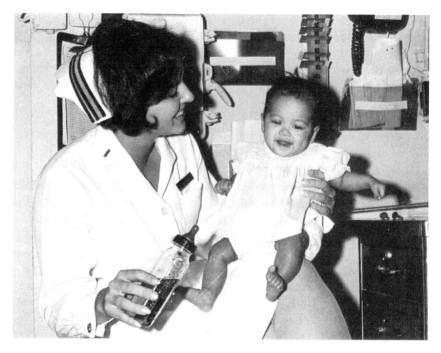

Ensign Anne Kuhn Gartner with Vietnamese orphan brought to ship for treatment. Note starched white uniform. Photo by permission.

had two female Red Cross workers on the ship that took care of all the patient's, hospital staff and ship's crew Red Cross needs, such as handing out toiletries, writing letters, and providing entertainment for the patients and staff.

On the ship there were about 30 female nurses and one female MSC officer. She was the blood bank officer, a very important job. She was also my roommate. There were usually two people to a room with two beds, two closets, two safes, and a sink. The bathrooms were down the hall. There was one room with three bunks. Basically, we all shared a room, as opposed to the ship, USNS *Mercy*, where you shared with eight others. The nurses had better quarters. We were also the only ship in the Navy to have a bathtub, a blue one. The nurses loved taking baths, but because of water rationing we had to conserve water. The nurses were mindful and used the bathtub sparingly! They put us on the top forward of the ship, right behind the two captains' quarters to "protect" us. The rooms weren't bad either. You had enough space. We wore the white uniforms and had a good laundry. We could wear civilian clothes when we were in our rooms or if they were having a picnic or party. Usually, we were in uniform. We were allowed to go up on one of the upper decks and sunbathe at specific times. The doctors and dentists were allowed up there with us, but not the enlisted.

The hospital had a 500-bed capacity, but could expand to 750 or 1,000 by opening the upper decks of the ship for less critical and ambulatory patients. We had about 200 corpsmen, 30 doctors, a few dentists, etc. Both of the current Navy hospital ships now are 1,000 without expanding. The *Sanctuary* only had four operating rooms. Now, they have 10 or 12. The hospital ships today have a much larger staff than the *Repose* or *Sanctuary*. Both the ships were converted oil tankers. The ship had a round

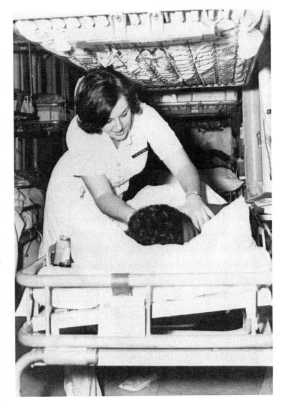

Ensign Anne Kuhn Gartner giving back rub to patient on the medical ward. Photo by permission.

bottomed profile. We were about half the length of the USNS *Mercy* or USNS *Comfort*. We had two complete crews. We had the crew for the hospital commanded by a captain. We had a line officer captain who was CO of the ship. We had a complete compliment of ship's crew and hospital crew. There was about 500 staff total that manned the ship.

When the *Sanctuary* was steaming off the coast, the *Repose* was offloading patients in Da Nang, which would last for about three or four days. Then the ships traded places. They would steam, and we would offload patients. When receiving patients, we got them at all times of the day or night. We would treat them directly from the field. They came in with all their gear, weapons, hand grenades, etc. They were brought onto the ship by helicopters, sent to the triage area, not far from the chopper pad, checked over by a master-at-arms, who made sure all the weapons were removed, triaged and sent down to the pre-op area. Patients went into surgery, back to the PACU, and then up to the ward. The acuity of most of the patients was critical. They came in with severe land mine injuries. Some would be triaged and managed in Marine hospitals at the front. But, if we got patients directly from the field, they had already been treated by a corpsman putting a tourniquet on or giving them morphine. We had a large ICU. The nurses that worked ICU were kept very busy.

We depended so much on our hospital corpsmen. They were so prepared and learned so much from the doctors and nurses. We expected a lot more from them than we do now. I think the corpsmen got better training. They were in corps school longer. They got more practical, clinical experience before they got mobilized. Nurses, today, don't get the same amount of clinical experience while students as we got. As senior students, the only thing we weren't allowed to do was carry the narcotics keys. We had great corpsmen on the ship. Sure, we had a few screwups, but they didn't last long in the clinical areas. If they didn't work out, they were sent to nonclinical areas, such as the laundry or mess hall. Another difference in nursing staff on the ship between Vietnam and Desert Storm may have been just the attitude about nurses.

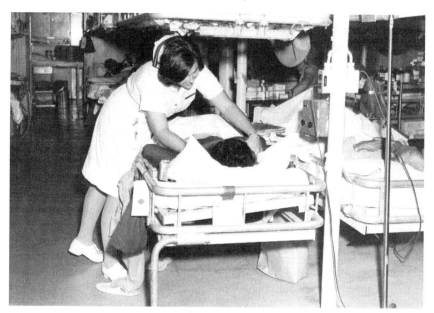

Ensign Anne Kuhn Gartner repositioning a patient on the bottom bunk on the medical ward; the sicker patients were on the bottom bunk. Photo by permission.

Nurse planners during Desert Storm realized that the nurses couldn't do everything for everyone and staffed with a lower nurse-patient ratio.

I spent my year on a ship. We had huge numbers of patients. One night we got 250 patients transported directly from the field. They all had immersion foot, caused because these men were not able to change their socks, shoes, or really take care of their feet. When they stomped around in the rice paddies with all that water, their feet just became swollen and horrible. We had to get them off their feet and treat the infection. On the *Sanctuary*, the medical wards were set up two, three or four bunks high. As your acuity improved you moved higher up because then you could get in or out of the upper bunks. Some of our wards, like our holding wards, you may have five bunks high. We had to move a lot of the patients from lower bunks to upper bunks to accommodate these Marines with immersion foot. We used the edge of the bunks to climb up and treat the patients. We all still wore white starched uniform dresses then. My Catholic mother said, "You can't be showing off your underwear." She had me wear these cute pantaloons with all this frilly lace on it. The guys got a good show of some nice lace. If you had to take care of a patient on the top bunk, you had to climb up there. It was different nursing. You learned to be pretty inventive and to really be able to assess what was going on very quickly.

You could get 20 or 30 patients at a time. They came from helicopters into Da Nang Harbor where the ship was anchored. Patients also came in by boat launch. They would be seen in triage and admitted to the ward. We would get a large influx of patients with malaria. We had a really good lab that looked at the malaria blood smears. You had to treat them by figuring out what type of malaria and then start them on the established treatment regime. Some of the corpsmen would learn how to read the blood smears, but the nurses just didn't have that kind of time. I did learn how to do a lumbar puncture. We had some very interesting cases. Because of where we were, the people were brought in from the rice paddies and the civilian populations. We got to see a lot of cases of diseases or injuries you might not see in a Stateside hospital.

The nurses bonded. You had to because you were always relying on someone else to come relieve you. If your shift was over and you had a huge influx of patients, nurses stayed. Where were you going to go? There wasn't a lot of places to go on the ship. You did need some down time. We did get off the ship and out to some of the tourist places. I also had an opportunity to do an exchange with an Army nurse at the 95th Evac in Da Nang. Let me tell you, that was an experience. The nurse that went off the ship didn't want to go back to the hospital because she had clean sheets, three square meals a day and people weren't shooting at her. It was an experience. You spent a lot of time under your bunk with your flak jacket and helmet on. Most of the guards on the perimeter were not Army soldiers. They were the corpsmen. They had to do their duty as Army medics and then go to the perimeter. I did get to travel in Vietnam to see the big caves with the beautiful Buddhas. We went into the Philippine port a number of times because we had to go into dry dock. We would spend five to seven days there. We also had two flights we were allowed to take, either to Hong Kong, Singapore or Japan. We had to go into Da Nang Airport to go on those R&Rs. When I came home, we were in the Philippines, so I flew home out of Clark Air Force Base.

This experience was a real immersion in the trauma that can happen in war. I think some of the nurses did well and some didn't. People had to realize that you had to be able to let go. You had to be able to go home at night and sleep and let go of the patients and what was going on around you. Some learned how to do it very well and some didn't. The ones that didn't adapt very well had a tendency to drink a lot. We didn't generally send them home. A couple went home early because of family issues. If you got pregnant, you were sent home. At that point in time, you were kicked out of the Navy. It had nothing to do with a moral judgment. Marriage and/or pregnancy were situations that kept you out of the service.

Why did I want to be stationed in Vietnam? That is a very good question. Navy nurses were stationed in three main locations in Vietnam: the two hospital ships *Repose* and *Sanctuary*, and NSA Da Nang Station Hospital. When I was stationed at Corpus Christi, Texas, I met three nurses who had been stationed on the *Repose* and got orders to Texas. I enjoyed listening to the stories of being a nurse in a war zone. I felt, with the experience I had gained from my brief civilian career in PACU and the experiences in Corpus Christi, Texas, a tour on board a hospital ship would be a very important addition to my career in military nursing. As a nurse, I was able to request orders to go to Vietnam. There were about 5,000 military women who served in Vietnam, 90 percent being military nurses. We had two Red Cross women volunteers who were on the ship. This was not true for most of the enlisted hospital corpsmen that were stationed on the ships or in Vietnam. The draft was still going on and most men did not have the option of not going to the war. This was also true for most of the enlisted Army, Marines and Air Force personnel. For these people, the last place they wanted to go was "in country" where the war was dangerous, up close and very personal. The hospital corpsmen that were assigned to the ships had it a bit better than those that were at the Station Hospital in Da Nang or in the field with the Marines as the medical care for the thousands stationed throughout the country of Vietnam. The corpsmen stationed with the Marines were such an important part of the treatment process for patients being transferred from the field to the ships and station hospitals and, eventually, Stateside. The Navy doctors and dentists stationed at the aid stations that provided medical support for the injured were instrumental in training the corpsmen in so many things that helped to stabilize patients before they were medevacked to more definitive treatment out of the battlefield.

Today I look back at the many experiences that I encountered in Vietnam. It was the foundation for my life in military nursing and my career in the future years. The most important was teaching and training the enlisted to function in the hospital setting and providing leadership for the junior personnel, both officer and enlisted. Not everything that transpired in the war was pleasant or easy to handle for a 20-year-old Navy nurse (I celebrated my 21st birthday in Vietnam) without a number of life experiences. War is not fun and things you see or experience can have a very profound impact on you for the rest of your life. Being stationed on the ship was a little safer that being "in country" but even the large red crosses painted on the side of the ship would not deter the enemy from trying to harm us. On Christmas Eve, the ship was anchored in Da Nang Harbor to offload patients and take on new ones. This was a normal part of our duties while the *Repose* was stationed up at the DMZ to take on patients for three or four days. It was after dinner and Catholic mass was being said up on the upper deck. All of a sudden, the ship was doing an emergency weighing of the anchor. We were under way to exit the harbor as quickly as possible. Then an announcement was made over the IMC that "swimmers" had been spotted coming toward the ship. We needed to be underway and back out into open water to prevent any military action against the ship. Because we were a hospital ship and had medical personnel under the Geneva Convention did not mean that the North Vietnamese always followed the rules. Also, there was a civilian hospital ship, treating civilian Vietnamese casualties, that was docked in Da Nang. Our ships' personnel were very aware of any activity of the ship preparing to leave the dock, in the event they were given a "heads up" about any hostile military activity that could harm them. That happened a couple of times when we were in Da Nang. Our ship would only anchor during the day, but not stay the night and would depart and steam in open waters until the "threat" was no longer apparent.

I had mentioned the hospital ships were converted oil tankers with round bottoms. After a night steaming in open water, the ship would pull into the harbor in early morning to anchor and take on supplies and patients and offload patients and other personnel. About 0630, heading into the harbor, I was just getting a report on the medical ward at the start of shift. All of a sudden, everyone knew something was not "right." The ship began listing to port and it was very difficult to stay upright. The patients in their bunks were screaming "grab on to something and hold on for dear life," which I did. But that was not the end of it. The ship hovered there for what seemed like an eternity. Then, we started to go back in the opposite direction. I could see out the door of the ward that the ship was going to do the same thing, but in the opposite direction. Then I saw sky and I was not sure what was going to happen. I was still holding on for dear life, praying at the same time, when the ship seemed to hover even longer in the starboard direction. I did not know what was going to happen. All of a sudden, we started to go back to upright. We were still rocking, but not as bad as the first two episodes.

That was such a very scary situation. The crew did not realize how serious until a few minutes later when an announcement came over the 1MC that the ship had hit a "surface wave" entering the harbor. The sea was calm, but right below the surface, there were waves that interfered with the ship's round bottom that caused us to rock dangerously to the port and starboard. If the ship had gone just a few more degrees to the starboard, we could have capsized. Thankfully, the ship's captain and crew were able to avoid the catastrophe. The hospital crew and ship's crew spent most of the morning picking up all the things that had been dislodged during the "event." We were so very lucky that everything worked out well. We later learned that the ship's captain "turned white" during the transit that day into the harbor.

Security was always a concern for the ship's personnel. Every patient that came aboard the ship, whether for admission or an appointment, was checked by the Master at Arms for any weapons which were removed and locked up in the "armory." When any medical personnel left the ship, we were also accompanied by some form of security, not so much in Da Nang, but if we went into other areas, we had armed Marines with us. You never knew who in the civilian population was armed or "booby trapped," even the children. When driving in Jeeps, you never left the road to make sure there were no land mines. We flew in helicopters to various locations. The chopper crews were also very aware of hazards and were very careful about landing, if there were any threats.

During the time I was in Vietnam, there were only a couple of times I was a bit scared. The first was the night I arrived in Vietnam at the station hospital and again, when I did the two-week trade at the 95th Army Evac Hospital in Da Nang. Being "in country" was a completely different experience than being on a ship. To tell the truth, most of the time we were so busy that we did not think about it as much as maybe we should have. That does not mean that we had not heard stories of what was happening in the field and some horrors of "fragging" officers by members of their squads or companies. It was not until I returned Stateside that I was really more aware of horrible things that happened in Vietnam. Being overseas, we were insulated from what was going on in the rest of the world, especially all of the protests of the war and unrest in the U.S. I know some crew members got letters from family and friends letting them know, but we did not talk about it. After serving my year on the ship, I received PCS orders to report for duty at Naval Hospital San Diego, California.

I departed the ship when the ship was in the Philippines for scheduled maintenance. I flew out of Subic Bay to Travis AFB in California. The trip was a lot shorter than the trip over. At that time, we flew in uniform. I was in my dress blues. We landed at Travis and bussed to San Francisco Airport for a flight home to Ohio for leave before I reported to San Diego. I started to notice that being in uniform attracted a lot of attention, but not the right kind. Lots of stares and sneers from some people. Most just ignored me. It was not until I got inside the airport and checked in for my flight that things changed. I found the gate for my flight to Ohio and started to walk in that direction. More people were giving me attention, some shouting at me. One even spit at me as I walked by. I was trying to remain calm and not let it bother me, but the farther I walked the more evident it became that I was not welcome wearing a military uniform.

I decided to find a pay phone and call my parents and let them know I was in the airport waiting to catch my flight home. It was so great talking to them on the phone and not over a radio or by reading a letter. I was so fortunate having such a supportive family and friends. After the phone call, I found a restroom. I went inside a stall and tried to become less "military." I took off the devices on my raincoat, took off my black tie and left my blouse open, took off my military cover, stashing it in my carry-on bag. I took off anything that looked like a uniform. I had very small heel shoes on but did not have another pair of shoes to change into so just left them on. I decided to take my wallet out of my military purse, put it in my raincoat pocket and put the purse in the carry-on. I wished I had a scarf to tie around my head, but I did not, so I had to go as I was. I waited until the restroom was empty, came out and looked in the mirror. I was completely dressed in black, but did not have anything military on. I walked out, proceeded to my gate and waited in a seat in the far corner of the gate waiting area until the flight boarded. I remember sleeping most of the flight home, so I did not have to interact with anyone on the plane. What a rude awakening from where I had been.

Once I got home, I had time to really start looking into what the mood of the country was while the war was still going on in Vietnam. It was in the paper and on the TV every night, so you soon became aware of the feeling of the country. Remember this was the early 1970s. My parents were so proud of my service to my country and what I had accomplished, but I did not feel that comfortable talking about my experiences in the airport. It was not until later, before I left for San Diego, that I talked about it. By then, I was getting excited about my next duty station, a new chapter in my life. I did talk to my mentor in Washington, D.C., when I was home. We talked about the situation. She told me that I handled it well. There would always be people who were against the war and took it out on any military, including the nurses, doctors and corpsmen that were there to provide care. I was glad to get back to a military hospital and a town that really supported the military: San Diego.

I was so fortunate to have support from the military family that I was a part of in the Navy. Most of my dearest and longest lasting friendships are those that I made in the military. I will always be proud of my military career. I did find it interesting that nurses at San Diego, who had not been in Vietnam or stationed overseas in direct support of patients right out of Vietnam, had a little different perspective on the war. I remember that a group of nurses were going to the movies to see the new movie *M*A*S*H*. I thought it was such a funny movie and really laughed during the whole thing, as it brought back experiences of being in a war zone. After the movie was over and we went out to eat, some of the new ensigns and lieutenant JGs seemed a little disturbed by my reaction to the movie. I said that life was so different in Vietnam.

We all had our own defense mechanisms to deal with what we saw, as patients were brought in straight from the battlefield. We all had to find coping mechanisms when we were there and had to maintain a "normal" life both at work on the wards and off duty. Being on a ship, there were not many places to go. You did the best to enjoy the friends you made and enjoyed activities when you had time off. Unless you have been in the situation, you might not understand completely. Getting off the ship to go to Da Nang or visit sites in Vietnam were our opportunities to lead a normal life. The ship also would go into Subic Bay for maintenance. It gave us a chance to go shopping at the exchange, or go swimming at the officers' club, or get our hair and nails done and enjoy meals at different places on and off base. We were able to wear "civilian clothes" and travel around the Philippines to see the country.

It was fun to see the country, interact with people and have an opportunity to see the arts and crafts that were made in the Philippines, especially the silver work, monkey pod wooden bowls and the beautiful fabrics they created. I still have the silver napkin rings and the napkins, but the "monkey pod bowls" did not survive the many moves in the military. Also, each person was able to take an R&R trip while stationed on the ship. I was able to go to Tokyo and Hong Kong during the year I was there. Both places were great for sightseeing, shopping and buying lots of items you might not be able to get Stateside. Things to buy: pearls in Japan and handmade clothing and jewelry in Hong Kong.

I am so fortunate to have had the opportunity to experience military nursing in Vietnam and would not have traded my time there for anything. My life and future have always been founded on the many experiences. Some were good and some bad, but you learn to deal with them and move on. I think I am a better person for having experienced them. I remember being in Washington, D.C., when the Vietnam Women's Memorial was dedicated on November 11, 1993. My husband and I traveled to march in the parade and be there during the dedication ceremony. While I was at the ceremony, a man came up to me and said, "I remember you. You were a nurse on the *Sanctuary* when I was a patient." He thanked me for taking care of him and really appreciated seeing the nurses at the memorial. What a wonderful thing to happen all those years later. I know many Vietnam vets do not want to talk about or remember what happened over there. I think for me, it is important to remember, but to respect those who do not want to relive those experiences.

Many years later, being a Vietnam vet was finally accepted and the war protests had faded. Now, when someone says, "Thank you for your service," I answer back, "It was my privilege and honor." I only wish we would have been greeted with "Welcome home" instead of the shouts, sneers and spitting that occurred to so many Vietnam vets.

After I finished up my tour in Vietnam, I got orders to San Diego. I spent 18 months there. I worked in the medical and surgical wards. Most of my time was spent working nights, which I loved. On the night shift you were much more independent. You weren't put on committees, and the parking was easier. I worked two weeks nights, had five days off, and then back again for another two weeks. I had four wards: two orthopedics, ENT, and urology. I had permanent corpsmen that worked the same schedule I did and it was great. One of the other nurses worked the same schedule in the ER. We would take off and go traveling. We learned that you have to change your whole schedule around in order to work permanent nights. We would eat our breakfast when we got up. When we got off work, we'd go eat our dinner. We really did not have a hard time adjusting to nights. I finally got a set of orders out of San Diego to go to Newfoundland, which I was happy about because I wanted more experience.

Right before I was ready to leave, I got another set of speed orders that said I wasn't going to Newfoundland. Someone who was scheduled to go somewhere else was now diverted to Newfoundland. The person who was supposed to go there can't go, and now you're going to Iceland. This happened because I put Iceland on my dream sheet many years ago. I loved Iceland. It was a very small station hospital with a small contingent of nurses and doctors. We had two operating rooms. The nurse anesthetist, who was the only anesthesia provider there, was responsible for all the stuff that happened in the OR. The nurse anesthetist there had to be sent back to the States due to a medical condition. They then sent a doctor, an anesthesiologist, up to do a TDY for a period of time. He could not run the OR. The head nurse wanted to know if there was anybody who was willing to run the OR. I knew CSR. He delivered babies up there, so it was not a big step to go from the labor room to the operating room. I had three outstanding HM2 corpsmen that were OR techs, who basically taught me everything I needed to know. I worked the OR the last six months I was there. I loved it. I met my husband when I was stationed in Iceland. I did a lot of traveling. The country of Iceland is beautiful. I traveled through Iceland and Europe. It was not a bad place to be stationed.

We did have an older hospital in Iceland. Eventually, a new hospital was constructed. It was a very close-knit family. There is a large Air Force contingent there. So, you got to know the Air Force people. You saw them at the clinics. You took care of their kids, husbands and wives. They also had an active sports group. We had a women's basketball league. We had a large teaching contingent because they had a DOD school there. The nurses and some of the wives of military members won the league championship against the teachers' team. It was cold there, sure, but we got used to it. I arrived in October when it was dark. I left in October when it was dark. It was like the ship. You learned to rely on each other.

We had squadrons of both Air Force and Navy P3s that came in. My husband was on one of the P3 squadrons deployed to the base and was the tactical coordinator with one of the crews. As the tactical coordinator, he was the officer that deployed the sonobuoys and listened to them to track Soviet submarines. We also were very fortunate that in Iceland we had a good working relationship with some of the hospitals in Reykjavik, the capital. We attended seminars with some of the nurses and tried to do things that made our educational opportunities better. We also had opportunities to take classes at the university on the base. You could do a lot when you were there. I was in Iceland from 1971 to 1972. I was looking for a place to go while dating my future husband. He was at Pax River, ~~New Jersey~~ *MARYLAND* and his squadron was transitioning down to Jacksonville, Florida. I couldn't get to Jacksonville, Florida, because they didn't have any billets available. My detailer said I could go to either Key West, Florida, or Beauford, South Carolina. I looked at a map and said, "Beauford is a lot closer than Key West."

I went to Beauford in October 1972. I was there less than a year because I got married the following January. The detailer said, "I'll give you no cost orders" to Jacksonville. It cost me about $350 to rent a truck and pack up all my stuff. Beauford, South Carolina, was a pretty small hospital. It was a large facility with many closed wards and not a lot of patients. The closest military base was Parris Island, the Marine training base. I got a lot of patients from there. There was also a large, retired population. Jacksonville was a good size teaching hospital and had all of the medical services. I started working outpatient clinics and the ER. I spent only about a year at Naval Hospital Jacksonville.

In 1973, I got out of the Navy. My husband and I were going to go back to school. I wanted to do something else. My husband had already gotten out. He didn't retire. He just got out. Being in aviation and nursing, it was difficult to get stationed together. We both stayed in the naval reserves. It was hard to get a billet in the reserves. I was very lucky to slide into a billet. It was for clinic work. We moved to Tampa, Florida, and both enrolled at the University of South Florida. Every month we'd drive up to Jacksonville and do our reserve duty. Jeff would fly and I would work at the reserve center taking care of the reserve personnel medical needs. We did that for about three years before we moved to California.

When I got out of the active Navy, I went back to college. I had never been to college, except for the year I took classwork for nursing school. I found there were opportunities for other careers. I found that I enjoyed the hard sciences like geology. I really did want to be a Marine biologist, but it would have taken another 13 years to get a Ph.D. I went on and got a degree in geology. I didn't work part-time while I was going to school because I did a lot of extra drills in the Navy. I would work at the clinic or the hospital. I kept up my skills and maintained my nursing license.

We moved to California after I got my bachelor's degree in geology in 1975. I was able to get a part-time job three or four days a week. I went over to the naval reserve to see what nurse billets they had. I was able to get a reserve nurse billet. I went to Naval Hospital Oakland, went up to the OR and told them I would like to work in the OR or volunteer my time. They said, "Oh, well you can do some of your drills here." Every Wednesday for four years I went to Naval Hospital Oakland and worked in the OR.

In the reserves we always had a joke that someday they're going to deploy everybody, leave the key on a hook, and the reserves are going to come in to staff the hospital. That is exactly what happened in 1990 with Desert Storm when I was recalled to active duty. I had been working in the OR plus I was selected as commanding officer of a number of naval reserve medical units. I was the senior nurse in the OR. There was one commander who was active duty who was not deployed to staff the USNS *Mercy*. She was appointed as the supervisor for the operating room and the PACU. But I was essentially running the OR. We were operating a full daily surgical schedule.

The war came along in August 1990. The day we got recalled, the nurses were attending a weekend Trauma Nurse Corps Course at the naval hospital. It was a Saturday when we got recalled by the reserve center and were told to report for active duty on Monday to Naval Hospital Oakland. We finished the course and were all mobilized.

I went right to Naval Hospital Oakland. That's where my reserve billet was assigned. The active-duty DNS at that hospital was deployed to the hospital ship. The active duty ADNS stepped in as the director of nursing service. In early September, I received a call in the OR. The XO and the commanding officer wanted to see me in twenty minutes. The secretary there said, "Oh, captain, just have a seat and they will be with you in a few minutes." I had moved up in rank from lieutenant commander to commander at Reserve Center Alameda when I was there as a reservist. I was on the promotion list for captain when I was mobilized, but didn't get to put on the stripe until December 1990.

I first saw the XO and CO. They were looking to replace the ADNS. They were interviewing a number of the captains who came in with the reserve contingent. There were no active-duty candidates because all of them had been deployed. A day or so later they called me up and asked me if I wanted the job. Of course, you're not going to turn that down. It was a very rewarding job. It showed the reservists could come in and put that hospital back into full operations and not miss a beat. We had personnel from all over the country including Alaska and Hawaii. We did have some major logistical problems. Bringing personnel in from all over, finding places for them to live and how they're going to get from point A to point B was challenging. I think we did a pretty good job of making it as bearable as possible. Lots of people were away from home and family. We did a very good job of becoming a functioning hospital in a very short period of time. The most difficult thing were all the rumors and disinformation. We didn't know very much about what was actually happening. Most of what we knew we got from CNN.

I stayed on as DNS until September 1991 when the active-duty DNS returned from *Mercy*. I transitioned into a billet as a special consultant. I did analysis of different medical programs and provided reports to better serve the needs of the patients and modernization of the hospital spaces. We were going through the reconstruction of the hospital. I remained on active duty for over 13 months. Then the hospital started getting all the medical personnel back that had been deployed on the *Mercy*. They came home, took their leave and we started releasing the recalled reservists. I think I was the last nurse corps reservist to leave.

I then was selected to be the REDCOM nurse and went back to my civilian job at the U.S. Geological Services (USGS). It was a tough transition back to civilian life. I had been concentrating on nursing for so long! All of a sudden, to come back to an entirely different job was difficult. It took about two and a half years to really get back to where I was before because it's so different. My career with USGS transitioned into other jobs. I did HR, science administration and management. I loved the research and geology work, but after being away for 13 months, I realized my strengths were more in management and administration. Running the directorate at the naval hospital gave me opportunities in budgeting, succession planning and FTE. In the long run, that was a very good position to be in and served me well during the remainder of my time in USGS. I'm very pleased with how things turned out.

When I became the REDCOM nurse, I was also selected as the only nurse in REDCOM 20 that was head of the entire medical department, usually held by a reserve physician. After I finished in REDCOM, I took over as the CO in the 1000 person medical unit assigned to Naval Hospital San Diego, even though I was living in San Jose, California. I traveled to San Diego four to five days each month to drill at the hospital. I was there three years before I retired in December 1999 with almost 32 years of military service. The reason I got out of the Navy was because I saw there were a lot of commanders and young captains that really needed to have the same opportunities that I had in my career. I felt I had served my country. I had done everything I wanted to do. I could have gotten another billet, but I felt it was important to let the new commanders and captains have the opportunities. I always felt your time comes and you have to move on. If you haven't done a good enough job teaching them so that they can take over, then you haven't done your job. I had a lot of good mentors during my career to help me get where I needed to be. I felt it was my time to give back.

In my civilian job I was the RMO (regional management officer) for the Geologic Discipline for eight different geology teams in California, Washington, Arizona, and Alaska up until October 1, 2007. After a reorganization, I became a SPO (science program officer) because of my geology background. I retired from federal service in January 2009 with 37 years of service.

Susan Searle Jackson

My grandmother, mother, and aunt were all nurses, but did not serve in the military. My mother wanted to be a military nurse, but she was considered mission essential, managing the operating room at a large teaching hospital affiliated with the University of Minnesota. She was a Red Cross volunteer nurse during World War II. She was also on the nursing faculty at the University of Minnesota. My father was in the Air Force. I chose to join the Navy because they had the best scholarships, at the time.

I graduated from high school in Farmington, Minnesota, in 1968. Today, Farmington is a suburb of the Twin Cities. At that time, it was a small town about twenty-five miles from the core of the city. Upon getting sound advice from my mother, I chose to go to the College of St. Catherine to get my baccalaureate degree in nursing. It also was a tradition for women in my family, aunts, cousins, to attend this college. I graduated in 1972.

The Vietnam War was going on during my high school and college years. Even at my college, an all-girls school, we had war protests and peace sit-ins to get out of Vietnam. It was not a popular time to think about a career in the military. When I was a sophomore, a Navy nurse recruited me. She was a graduate of my college and one reason I joined. Another reason was that during my sophomore year I was working as a nurse's aide at one of the big hospitals. A weekend ward clerk happened to be a corpsman in the recruiting office. Between the two of them, they just kept giving me information. Finally, I thought, "This is silly not to take advantage of this opportunity." I didn't dare discuss that idea with any of my peers at college. It just was not something that you thought about back then because of the Vietnam War. I did come home and showed all the papers to my mother. She was very supportive of the idea and thought it would be a good idea to join.

As a Navy Nurse Corps candidate, the Navy paid for my junior and senior year of college. That included tuition, books and a stipend.

Considering that I needed money to pay for school, it was a tremendous opportunity. It was different than ROTC because there were no military drills and I didn't wear a uniform. I just attended school like any other nursing student. I worked at a local hospital. The Navy gave me a nurse corps candidate pin, of which I was very proud and put it on my student nursing uniform. Even though the war was going on, I still wore that pin. My instructors and my nursing classmates did comment on it.

My senior year, three other nursing students became nurse corps candidates. We graduated in May and immediately reported to Newport, Rhode Island, for Officer Candidate School (OCS). I had never been in New England. I was looking forward to everything I had heard about Newport. It wasn't the easiest of times. You were learning everything about the Navy. They were very strict about inspections. We had exams almost every day. I did really well. I graduated at the top of the class as a distinguished graduate.

OCS was six weeks long and you transitioned from civilian to military life. The hardest part for me was passing the swim test. I am not a strong swimmer. I had to go in for extra remedial swimming and strength training. They took me to the top of this diving board and told me to jump off with my clothes on, and inflate my pants to make it like a life preserver. I could not look down. I knew when I walked down that diving board, if I looked down, I would never do it. I just walked off the board. I weighed 90 lbs. When I hit the water, the impact knocked the breath right out of me. But I passed the swimming test. I wasn't really into physical fitness. I didn't run or jog. We had to complete an obstacle course and lots of marching. I would say all of the physical exercise was the most difficult for me at Newport. We first attended class in civilian clothes, then finished by wearing military uniforms. I was in the very first company, Company D, that had a male instructor.

Here is a funny story. In 1972, females were endorsing bra burning in the USA. Some girls at OCS were not wearing bras. Our male company instructor had to get up in front of our company, before the uniforms came, to say that the bra was part of the uniform and that it needed to be worn at all times. I'm sure they had to do that in every company. Years later, I got to be good friends with our instructor. I asked him if he remembered that incident. He said, "Oh my gosh, I sure do." It was one of the most embarrassing things that he had to say. Today that would be considered sexual harassment or you would put it in writing in a memo. It would say, "You must read this memo and sign it."

In Newport, you were assigned to a buddy at your first duty station. Mine became a lifelong friend. I still see her all the time. The duty station that I was assigned was Great Lakes, Illinois. At first, I was disappointed that I didn't get assigned near the ocean, the East or the West Coast. My recruiter said, "Oh, this is a fabulous teaching hospital." For me, a kind of shy person, I had some friends that were going to be in the Chicago area at civilian hospitals. I had an aunt and uncle that didn't live far away. I could get home to Minnesota. So, I thought, "As long as it is a very large teaching hospital, it still will be a big adventure going there and living near the big city of Chicago. I guess this will be okay for my first duty station." And, it was.

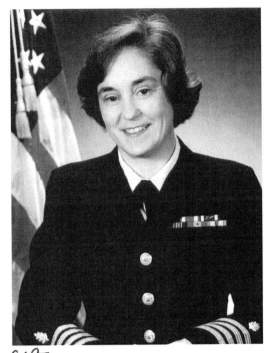

CAPT, LCDR Susan Searle Jackson. Susan served during the Vietnam era, the 9/11 crisis and Operation Desert Storm. Photo by permission.

As soon as I finished at Newport, I went home. I could not take my State Board of Nursing exam in Minnesota because it was given while I was in Newport, Rhode Island. I was assigned to take the exam in Illinois. I spent two weeks with my family and studied for the exam before reporting to Great Lakes Naval Hospital. Another girl and I drove the morning of the Illinois State Board Exam to central downtown Chicago. I had never seen a five-lane expressway and accidentally missed our exit. It was just awful. We had to find the convention center where the exam was given. We finally made it there with just minutes to spare. They let us in and till this day I just can't believe that I was calm enough to pass that exam. It was really something. I have never seen so many nurses in my life. The exam was two days long. We were able to calmly go to the other girl's house, which was in a suburb of Chicago. The next day we did a better job of getting there. That was my first real experience with big city traffic.

Both of us passed. We were very happy about that. I finished a brief nursing internship program and stayed in the postoperative recovery room. They also assigned me to work in the ICU. They just had a single ICU. That was early in the days of ICUs. There was no such thing as a central line. Swan-Ganz catheters came after I left the ICU. It was nothing like an ICU today. The nurse-patient ratio was less and another difference was the quality and level of education of the corpsmen. If you were a conscientious objector, you could choose to be a corpsman and serve in the military. The corpsmen assigned to the ICU all had college educations. One even had a master's degree in physiology. They were very smart and had unbelievable talent.

At five feet, one inch, and weighing 90 lbs. I was very small for a nurse. The scrub gowns we were given to wear in the ICU were always too big. They didn't have pants. The dress would go down to my ankles. I took them home, cut them off, hemmed them, and then I had to launder my own scrubs if I had any hope of keeping them. It was a funny time.

There were a couple of landmark changes that took place while I was at Great Lakes. Shortly after I got there, the Department of Defense came out with an announcement that if you were pregnant you didn't have to get out of the Navy. For the first time you were allowed to stay in. I remember the nurse that was in charge of a big medical ward became pregnant. There was no military uniform for her to wear. But, because of scrubs, she came to work with me in the recovery room. Pregnant nurses could also be assigned to central supply or sterile process, some place you couldn't be seen. Sometimes you worked the night shift. You had to become invisible. There was no official Navy uniform. That came a couple of years later.

Another thing that happened was that the Vietnam War ended. They were winding down the war in the fall of 1972. Great Lakes was one of the hospitals where they flew home some of the POWs in February 1973. Several of them came there. My roommate was chosen to work with them. I think you had to have a really bubbly personality. It was an exciting time at my hospital. Because the war ended, they made a decision that they were going to decrease the number of teaching hospitals for the physicians. Great Lakes was downsized. When all the doctors graduated on 1 July 1973, many of the big teaching programs ended. Great Lakes was no longer considered a big tertiary hospital. The change was pretty profound.

Great Lakes was still the main site for corps school. Later, they opened schools in Orlando and San Diego. There were also other enlisted schools. I know they were very worried about it. If you didn't have all the surgeries and residents, you didn't necessarily have all the patients for the corpsmen to take care of.

I remember the war before the POWs came back during that summer and fall. We would just get announcements that said, "Air evac arriving from O'Hare Airport." A bus would arrive and all the injured would be on it. They would call ahead and give you an idea about the injuries. We were prepared, working in the ICU, for critically injured patients to come. Patients were usually ages 18 to 22. The other thing I witnessed was the reaction of friends and family to the returning POWs. Often, it was the first time a girlfriend or family member saw the permanent injury or loss of a limb.

I remember our charge nurse. She was seasoned. She had worked on a hospital ship in Vietnam. It was tough love. Her philosophy was, "If you are upset, don't show it in front of the patient. Go to the side. I'm always there to talk to you. Put on a face for the patient and make them do their self-care as much as possible. Don't do everything for them because they are going to be this way for the rest of their life. They have to realize right now that they have to take ownership of their care. They have to have a positive attitude toward rehab." It would start right there in ICU. We were kind and helpful. We cared about pain, but we didn't exactly make it easy. If they were ambulatory, they had to go down to the chow hall. When vital signs were taken, we made the patients walk to the nursing station, no matter how much they cussed us.

The direct contact I had with injured veterans from Vietnam was when covering the hospital as the duty nurse for the evening and night tours. I remember that some veterans had sleep issues, so it was not unusual to see a patient sitting with a corpsman at the nurses' station in the middle of the night. I now know that PTSD was prevalent, but that was a medical diagnosis that I had never heard during the Vietnam era.

The hospital medical, surgical and orthopedic units were all set up as open bays. Only a curtain separated the patients. I think this actually helped patients to heal because they never felt alone. Nursing supervisors cautioned us not to let injured veterans stay in bed with closed curtains.

We had train tracks across from the hospital. We had a really bad accident where some guys in a car were trying to outpace a train and got hit. Two died. We were able to save two of them. They were all stationed on our base. I will never forget that call when it came in. I can remember how horrific it was. We just didn't see that kind of trauma. We weren't a "Cook County" type trauma center. To be taking care of your own people was very traumatic.

Another thing that happened was a little tornado hit a trailer park on base. We got some injuries. There were broken bones and some serious injuries. I had been on my way to work when that happened. I actually saw the funnel. It was the only time in my life I have ever seen anything like that. I knew what it was because you could see boards and things spinning around in it. There was another car in front of me. We just all stopped. It was further down the street. It went perpendicular to us. We thought, "Oh maybe it wasn't that bad." But, when we got to work, we realized it had hit the trailer park.

I was in the ICU/recovery room for nine months. Then, I requested a transfer to pediatrics. I was summoned to the office of the chief nurse. I can't tell you how scared you are when someone says, "When you finish your shift, you have to report to the chief nurse." Everything is going through my mind wondering how many mistakes I had made. I wasn't sure I could do it. I went to her office. She said, "They're going to outfit the hospital ship USS *Sanctuary* to be a dependents support ship. They will have pediatrics and they need a pediatric nurse who can speak Spanish." I had taken Spanish in college. I was not fluent. I had put on my dream sheet that I would like to work on a hospital ship. She asked me to go. Of course, I said "yes." Instead of completing my first two years at Great Lakes, I left early. I got to Great Lakes in July 1972 and left in September 1973. I had heard accounts of duty aboard the ship from nurses serving off the coast of Vietnam. I wanted that experience.

The ship was in Alameda Harbor, San Francisco, California. The ship had come home from Vietnam. It had been at the shipyard at Hunter's Point at San Francisco. There it was changed from this troop support ship, taking care of combat injuries, into a floating hospital for the fleet. It would be stationed in Greece. That was Admiral Zumwalt's idea. A huge factor was that the troops were so far away from their families. He hoped to bring the families to them and the ship could dock off Greece. It would go out on missions in the Mediterranean and the Persian Gulf. He felt that this would be better for morale.

The ship had been moved to Alameda. I had never been to San Francisco. Now, I was finally going to get to the ocean on a hospital ship. I was going to Greece. I cannot tell you how excited I was. They said, "Before you do that, they want to test this ship. So, the ship is going on a goodwill mission to Central and South America for a month. You will be the pediatric nurse on the ship. It will be like Project Hope, providing humanitarian services to the local population." I was permanently assigned to the ship at the end of September 1973.

Before going on the goodwill mission, the ship went on a training exercise from San Francisco to San Diego to get donated medical supplies, load up the ship and come back to San Francisco. A week later we began the long trip. I still remember going under the Golden Gate Bridge. It was a perfect day. We were manning the rails, as we went under the bridge. It was like you picture out of a movie. You can't believe you are really on this ship. There was a tradition that you were allowed to toss a coin into the ocean and make a wish as you went under the bridge. On this trip, we were allowed to design a special uniform. We decided on black pants and a white blouse. It wasn't the white nurses' pant suit. The pant suit was put in uniform inventory after we came back from the goodwill mission. It was a big deal when it was announced. When we came back, we were allowed to order the new pant suit. We didn't wear the salt and pepper look.

For the goodwill mission, we sailed down around Mexico. We didn't have many port stops. We were always at sea. We went to Buena Ventura, Colombia. It was very poor. We were there a month to provide health care to the local poor population. We opened clinics and did have two wards to keep some patients overnight. For the most part, care was ambulatory and only the people we did surgery on stayed overnight. Also, we made trips to little clinics in the village itself. It was unbelievable the patients we saw. These were poor people that came from the rural area. Word had been put out through their health system that the ship was there with supplies and medicine. They could see doctors. People came that had never seen a doctor. I remember seeing gigantic hernias. We had a plastic surgeon who performed cleft palate repairs on little babies. It was really heartwarming. Medically, we were always treating for parasites. I know they did other things on people with tumors. You did see things from poverty and malnutrition, like rickets. Surgical procedures were life-changing experiences.

I worked with a wonderful doctor who spoke fluent Spanish. Patients and families loved him. It was a really positive time. They asked me to teach giving antibiotic injections. In Colombia, you could just go to the drug store and buy an antibiotic. It was usually the father, the head of the household, who would give the injections. That was the first time in my life that we had to learn on the ship how to sterilize glass syringes and check needles on gauze to see if they had burrs on the end of the needles. They reused them. Everything was disposable at Great Lakes, but not in Colombia. It was older seasoned nurses that helped us review use of these reusable supplies. One of these nurses was an operating room nurse. She gave us classes on how to reuse gloves, how to see if there is any puncture. We could have told them how to do it with disposable supplies, but the Colombians would never have had disposable supplies. It was so unique. We had to teach the fathers in the household because "that was their role" if someone was sick. They had to give the antibiotic. We did a lot of immunizations on the ship, not as much preventive care as you would think.

People were so generous and grateful. They invited us to cultural events off the ship. We took day trips to Bogotá and Cali. The enlisted were very happy in that country because the people were very friendly and the dollar was strong. You got two to one. You could go to a really fancy restaurant and get a really nice meal at little cost. You had to be careful. The water wasn't good. You did have to worry about things like kidnapping and the drug cartel. Cali was where the cartel was. We were all warned. There were lots of classes about that.

In the ward room, all meals were formal. We were served by stewards, usually Filipinos. Every week we were given one linen napkin to use all week. We had one silver napkin ring with our name on it that we put away in a little cubby hole when we finished our meal. The XO was the president of the officer mess. We had to pay for our meals. There was a designated time that you came in for each meal. You sat, ate and were dismissed by the XO. If all officers were there, there would be a second sitting for the ensigns and LTJGs. We sort of liked that because you could be more yourself. You could tell jokes and laugh and be loud. When you were at the other sitting with the senior people, we sat according to rank. If there were a whole bunch of people missing, we were allowed to close up the gap. We were allowed to sit next to each other instead of next to an empty space. If you couldn't get there on time for a meal, you ate in the galley. I liked to do that, if I was on duty. The stewards would give you some of the food that they ate in the Philippines, lumpia and rice dishes. Enlisted went to the cafeteria style chow hall while officers ate in the wardroom. Today, all ship's crew eat cafeteria style.

I met my future husband in the ward room when I was assigned a seat next to him because we had the same date of rank. He was the electrical engineer and worked in the engine room. Over the time of the cruise, I became really fond of Bard. When we were in Colombia, I would go out with him in town, if he didn't have ship duty or quarterdeck and engine room watches. The clinic I worked in was mainly in the daytime, but sometimes I would have to do ward duty, too. We all took turns working the wards.

This uniform was different from when the ships were in Vietnam. During the Vietnam War, the women just had to wear a dress. You had lots of ladders on the ship. So, it was nice to be able to wear a pant suit. The other thing that was important about the *Sanctuary*, at this time, was that it was the very first ship in the Navy to have women line officers. There was a lot of publicity about it. The commanding officer on the ship was hand selected because of his willingness to have women on board. There were women in all areas: officers, chiefs, enlisted, deck hands and engine room technicians. I'm not going to say there weren't problems with the integration of women for the very first time. If you were pregnant, you didn't sail. There was the same thing with fraternization. There was inappropriate behavior between men and women in departments on the ship. Female berthing could be a problem. One enlisted chief had a very difficult time because there was no sleeping space for her in the chiefs' area. They put her with the enlisted. It was not good for her. She was older. This was her last duty before getting out of the Navy.

After we sailed from Colombia, the ship went through the Panama Canal. We had many visitors on board. It took one whole day to go through the Canal. We had a wonderful picnic celebration with food and a band playing. It was fabulous to go through the Canal. I thought, "Oh my gosh, I'm doing this. I've read about this my entire life and here I am going through." What I remember the most after we got through the canal was how choppy the Atlantic Ocean was in comparison to the Pacific Ocean. I never got seasick on the Pacific. Here we were in the Atlantic, sailing to Haiti and I thought, "You're immune to this." That was where I realized, "Maybe I'm not so immune." There was this pitching up and down and sideways. All I wanted to do was stay in my state room and bury my head. All we had was Dramamine. We had this little rule that if you were on duty, you couldn't take Dramamine. You had to be alert. It was the old thing of going out on the deck and throwing up over the side or going to the bathroom. I just remember feeling so seasick at first. I wasn't the only one. Other people were sick, too. It was a big difference between the Pacific and the Atlantic. My husband never got seasick. I think the first day was the worst. It was a real shock. I just thought, "Oh turn me around. I want the Pacific again."

The ship went to Haiti, Port-au-Prince. This country was unbelievably poor. What struck you was the corruption of the government. You had the few wealthy and a multitude of poor residents. In between, you had some people who worked for the government, this special middle class. They could get things. The majority of the people had nothing. They had prepared us about how different this country was going to be from Colombia. We were reminded that we were in Haiti as their guests. As much as we might not like something, their humanity and the things we saw there, this was the way it was. We were there to provide humanitarian care. There were some local LPN nurses that came on board ship to act as interpreters.

We were welcomed by the Haitian government. I went to some clinics in Port-au-Prince. I also had the unique experience of going out in the jungle on a helicopter. The helicopter landed in the field. We offloaded supplies and set up a temporary clinic. The local people came to us. We went to orphanages to do immunizations. We ran all of clinics on the ship. I was assigned to pediatrics again. We did a lot of teaching in the villages. When you went by the president's palace, you saw guards all around them. We were told not to stop to take any pictures because we would be confronted.

When we were in local hospitals, their operating rooms were open at the top. They weren't sealed. There were flies coming and going. It was very hot there. I remember they also reused supplies such as gloves and needles. Their urinary catheter system was open. The tubing went to an open can or jar instead of a sealed drainage bag.

We brought donated bassinets from some American hospitals to leave in Haiti. We planned to give them to the local hospital to use with sick neonates. We would see these little premature babies and your heart just went out to them. You wanted to help and give them everything. We found the bassinets could not go there. They were reserved for the wealthy who could pay or the government people who were special. The poor weren't special and couldn't have the bassinets. The first lesson I learned about foreign governments was that bribery was part of their culture, the thing that they know. If you want something, you have to bribe officials. It is not something in our culture. They did not consider it stealing if you set something down. They assumed you didn't want it and it was up for grabs. An example of this was that you could set down a blood pressure cuff, a stethoscope, any little thing and turn your back for a second and it might be gone. If you could catch them right away and asked them, they would give it back to you. We lost equipment right and left because our staff didn't understand that you couldn't set something down and take your hand off it or it would just walk away. These people were so grateful for any care that they received. They were extremely disappointed if you didn't give them something during their exam at the clinic. We went through vitamins like you could not believe. This made them very happy.

We would go to the orphanage run by the chaplain. We would bring doctors who would screen all the kids. We would decide if there was anyone who really needed to have surgery or was seriously ill. We would get permission from their parents or the orphanage to bring the children back to the ship for care. One child had a chicken bone stuck in his throat. He couldn't speak. He would make a croaking sound. We brought him back and did the surgery. This child was so emaciated. We kept this little boy on the ship so he could gain some weight and eat better. Everybody felt really good about it.

One time I went out on that helicopter to the Albert Schweitzer

Clinic way out in the middle of Haiti, voodoo country. When we landed, women came out and put the supplies in boxes or large baskets and carried them on the top of their heads. Standing very erect, they balanced the baskets without using their hands. They walked quite a way from the helicopter to their clinic with our supplies. The men would be watching, playing the drums. When we got to this clinic, there was no electricity and there were open windows without screens. You had to use the daylight. We had dentists, doctors, nurses and a lab tech to draw blood. There were over 200 people lined up to come to the clinic. These were people who had really bad abscesses. The dentists were only able to do extractions. Their teeth were so bad and there was no way to do fittings. Everybody was examined and arrangements made for a couple of people to come back to the ship for surgery.

I remember one lady, in particular. She had a huge abdominal tumor. You saw goiters and infections. In one little section of the clinic, they tried to do some local incisions and drainage of small abscesses. With others, they made arrangements to bring them back to the ship. When it got dusk, we loaded up on the helicopter and flew back to the ship.

The ship's home port was changing from Alameda, California, to Mayport, Florida. That was the whole reason that a humanitarian mission could be done. They thought the mission would be good publicity for the Navy and would test the ship.

While we were in Haiti, we got news that there had been a coup in the Greek government. The United States could no longer assign a fleet to Greece. The whole concept changed for this ship. It was very disappointing. When we got to Mayport, they didn't know exactly what they were going to do, but that the ship would serve as a dispensary right there in the port next to the ships of the fleet. Instead of everyone having to go to the dispensary in Mayport or Jacksonville Naval Hospital, sick call could be held and some small procedures could be done in the operating room, while they figured out what to do next.

This ship had been completely renovated. Now, what did the Navy want to do? The ship was decommissioned in February 1974. We felt like Santa Claus because we gave away an unbelievable number of surgical instruments. We had doctors come and say, "I dreamed about having this instrument and here you have it." Instead of wrapping up surgical instruments and putting them in storage, we gave away as much as we possibly could. This ship was outfitted with the best equipment. You felt kind of good that you had made some people happy, but it was sad to be packing up the ship and never being able to do the mission that you wanted to. They put the ship in mothballs in Philadelphia, then put it on the James River. Eventually, a church group bought the ship, and towed it to Baltimore.

I married Bard Jackson on July 27, 1974. We had a military wedding in the base chapel in Mayport, Florida. I had one female attendant, my best friend from home. We had six side boys making an arch with the swords. They were all officers that served aboard our ship. The chaplain on the ship performed the ceremony. We made the *Navy Times*, because it said, "SHIP MATES TIE THE KNOT." There was a real human-interest story here and a good way to publicize the officers' club. It was a fun wedding with all the people on the ship.

I got out of the Navy at the end of February 1975 and joined the reserves. I didn't always have a pay billet. I drilled for non-pay and retirement points except for the paid two weeks of active duty. Like everything in the reserves, over time everything changed. All of a sudden there was a change so that all doctors and nurses got paid.

I had different opportunities to go on active duty. About 1986, they were designing the new fleet hospital program. It would be a modern-day M*A*S*H tent hospital. The hospitals would be alike for the Army, Navy and the Air Force. In putting this hospital together, somebody found the standard operating procedures for the USS *Sanctuary*. My name was on it as one of the authors. I had helped write it as a collateral duty. I was asked if I would like to come on active duty for six months and help write the procedure manual for this fleet hospital. It was an interesting opportunity.

After the manual was written, 1988, they set up a permanent training place for the fleet hospital at Camp Pendleton. They have classes to learn all about the fleet hospital. I went as a nurse inspector for the initial class. It was a wonderful experience that lasted 17 days. A huge active-duty group from Long Beach, San Diego and Camp Pendleton came there. They tested the whole system, including mock patients. I did an evaluation, wrote it up and submitted a report.

I went on active duty when the nurse corps redid the billet specifications for nurses. The director of the Navy Nurse Corps said to me, "I want Navy nurses to be treated with respect, the same as the line officers." That is never going to happen if we use titles like "charge nurse" or "patient care coordinator. We are going to be like the line. We are going to be staff nurses, division officers, department heads and directors. Condense the job descriptions. We need to say what the minimum education and experience level is. We want to describe some billets that require doctorates."

Email didn't exist then. I made calls and sent out packages. It was an enormous amount of paperwork. I learned a tremendous amount from that project that helped me throughout the Navy. I learned that "No" just means the beginning of negotiations. If you are going to do something, don't do it real small because it will be overly analyzed. Think big. Submit at the deadline, not in advance. If you submit it early, you will be writing the document over and over again.

At that end of that experience, Desert Storm began. I had five years of experience teaching nursing, leadership and organization at Catholic University. I was asked to head up the nursing education programs at Bethesda Naval Hospital. We asked the reservists the very first day who was CPR certified. Less than half the hands went up. Immediately we had to do a marathon on that. Then we asked who had worked in the hospital and actually taken care of patients. It wasn't many hands. In the enlisted group, nobody had. They were HM2s older than 25, very mature with good civilian jobs that paid much better than military pay. Many of them were taking terrific pay cuts during mobilization. We said to them, "We need you. There will be nurses there to teach you clinical skills. There are procedure books. If you don't know how to do something, do not be embarrassed or ashamed. Just ask somebody. We are not on any kind of ego trip. We are going to all learn this together."

The amazing thing was, just because of their maturity and more confidence, the best patient care was given. We were supposed to ramp up slowly. Immediately, when patients were seen in the clinic they started admitting to the hospital. There was no ramp-up time. It was almost full throttle within a week. Doctors, nurses and corpsmen were focused on doing a good job. They talked and listened to the patients. They didn't have any of those little personal things that might happen to make it more difficult on the job. Quality indicators that you use to measure care just didn't show any problems. I stayed long enough to see the troops come back from the Gulf.

When the active-duty personnel came back, they were very disappointed that the hospital ran as well as it did. For example, in the operating rooms, on the civilian side, nurses were used to a rapid turnaround. You only get paid for the time you are doing a case. Reservists came in and changed things radically. Operating rooms became much more efficient. Reservists started a same day surgery program. We had a couple of nurses that were very experienced with it. They came in and said, "No, no, you don't have the patients go to different places. You have the patients come to one location for labs, x-rays, etc." They set up this whole same-day surgery area as a one-stop program. They just did a lot of small things that were long lasting changes. They were pretty important things, but sometimes they involved major moving of compartments.

For example, we had a person in charge of neurology-neurosurgery. He insisted that his neurology patients have their own six bed ICU next to his neurology ward. They couldn't be mixed with the other ICUs. The first thing that happened was that this physician was sent to the *Mercy*. The commanding officer at Bethesda gave permission to consolidate all the ICU beds in one area. We are going to have these people crossed trained for each other so that we have better coverage. When the active-duty staff returned, after three months, in the Persian Gulf, the deed was done.

Here is another lasting observation. Sometimes, long turnovers or transition periods with active duty may not necessarily be the best thing. There was no chance for a turnover or transition period with Desert Storm. You came in and did the best you could. You looked with eyes wide open, using common sense logic. You asked, "Is this best for the patient? Is this the way we want it? We have nothing to lose here. You can't fail if you try some new things. We have to provide safe quality care for the patient. It doesn't necessarily have to be the way that you found it." I think because of that there were a lot of new things tried. We had permission from top leadership to try new strategies. The director of nursing service was fabulous. She would say, "Let's give it a try. If it doesn't work, we just go back to the same way we've been doing it." I learned a lot from that time period. It was wonderful. That was the beginning of when the reservists truly were integrated with active duty. From that time on, I think it didn't matter where you were. They realized we could all work together. They realized that we all have things to offer each other. We learned a tremendous amount from the active duty about the military side of care.

Irma Klaetke

I GRADUATED FROM Cass Technical High School in Detroit, Michigan, in 1951. I went on to the four-and-a-half-year program at Wayne State University College of Nursing. I was in the program from 1951 to 1956. Wayne State College of Nursing was associated with and got experience at ten different facilities. These were major hospitals, public health, visiting nurse, and rural nursing each for a month. In my Navy career, I had ten different duty stations. For some reason, it seemed that very diversity I received in my College of Nursing back in Detroit stood me in good stead with all my duties in the Navy Nurse Corps.

I went on to Detroit Receiving Hospital, a very progressive and fine hospital. It had a huge emergency room area with 12 or 13 different rooms in the emergency section. While I was there, one of my friends had been in the Navy Nurse Corps for five years. She had gotten out of the corps and stayed with the reserves. I talked to her about the fact that I was ready for a change. I wanted to be exposed to different types of nursing, life experiences and education opportunities. I had been at Detroit Receiving for three and a half years. I went down to see the Air Force and the Navy Nurse Corps recruiters. I chose the Navy and came into the corps in 1960. I felt it was an opportunity to serve my country, have new life experiences and have opportunities for adventure and travel.

I went to Newport, Rhode Island, for officer indoctrination. I was in the sixth class of Women Officers' School. I did not always do so well with my academics and did not get liberty every weekend. It was hard to go back to studying after four and a half years of nursing school. I had trouble marching. One time, I nearly marched my company into the wall. It was quite an experience.

My first duty station was St. Albans, New York. I was there from 1960 to 1962. I was primary staff on the surgical wards, general surgery, SOQ and coverage for the recovery room. One thing that was so wonderful at St. Albans was the commanding officer on the weekends

127

would make rounds. He would come to every ward and talk to the nurse and the corpsmen and some of the patients. When you have weekend duty you are usually understaffed. Things don't always run as smoothly as you like. A little crisis may come up here and there. Whenever I had weekend duty, I looked forward to seeing him come through. Just that type of thing, in a senior person, has stayed with me all these years.

Many times, the supervisor on duty would come through. One time, I was making beds on SOQ. The supervisor from the operating room came through. She started helping me make this bed, then asked me how many more had to be taken care of. To have somebody, such as a lieutenant commander or commander, come through and help you with those duties or say "hi" and "thank you" was just such a wonderful feeling.

From 1962 to 1964, I was on MSTS (military sea transportation service) E.D. Patrick, a USSN ship. There were USS ships, which were strictly military. The staff and the crew were all military. On my ship, we had a military complement of about thirty people. The rest were Merchant Marines. We had the military staff, line officers such as CO, XO and supply officer. The rest were the medical department. In the medical department, we had two doctors, one of them brand new to the service, a hospital corpsman chief, a first class, a second and several third classes, two hospital corpswaves, and one hospital nurse—me. In the medical department there were 12 or 13 people. We had a 44-bed hospital on the ship and one operating room. We had a separate section for sick call for the women and children at one end of the hospital. At the other end were men and boys.

We transported troops: Army, Navy and Marine Corps. We transported retired people and dependents back and forth in the Pacific. Some of the time, it was so families could be with their servicemen, or because the dependents had to come back to the States. Some of the time it was for families to meet their military counterpart in these other countries. Routes included the ports of Hawaii, Japan, Korea, Philippines, Okinawa and Guam in various combinations. The ship left from Oakland Supply Center. We had a medical department in the Presidio, where we had a senior nurse and a senior medical commanding officer of the medical department. There were five ships in both the Pacific and Atlantic. Some of them were USS. Some were USSN. At one point, we went down to San Diego and picked up a thousand Marines who had completed boot camp about two weeks before. We got underway with these young men who had been home on leave with families and friends. Some had been infected with German measles. We activated the whole hospital. We had one sergeant who had mumps. We isolated him in an isolation room. That was one of the big experiences while I was on the ship.

When I had been on the ship for about five months, we had two surgeries at sea. That is quite an experience because the ship is rolling and listing and pitching. The new doctor we had aboard had a little trouble with seasickness. He was new in the service and new on a ship for only a few months. He was giving anesthesia. The other doctor was doing the surgeries, both appendectomies. I had an OR tech that was out of school from Oakland. I was circulating. Both of the young men walked off the ship recovered.

On the ship, we'd get to Hawaii and unload patients, troops and cargo. We would have liberty the rest of that day and overnight. The next morning we'd go on to Japan and the same thing would happen. In each port, except for Korea, we'd have an overnight. If everything

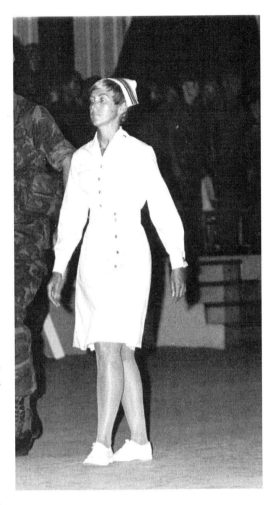

Lieutenant Commander Irma Klaetke leaves to join the crew of the USS *Repose*. It was Irma's second tour of sea duty with the "white shoe Navy." Photo by permission of George Klaetke.

was okay, we'd have liberty at that time. By the time we got back to Oakland, 33 days had passed. Then we'd have the weekend in port. I had a stateroom on the ship and stayed at the BOQ on Treasure Island. I had my car there. Another officer I was going with took care of my car. The manager of the club was retired Navy, so I was able to have my car parked there where it was pretty secure. While I was in Oakland, I had an apartment there.

On ships like the *Patrick*, the state rooms were set up for two to six passengers. There was a lounge area, and an auditorium that served as a chapel for Sunday services. It served as a movie theater and sometimes for passenger briefings. We also had a room where the chaplain and I had Sunday school for the children. There was a dining room and purser office because there was some kind of stipend that the retired people and the other people might pay to travel on this ship. There was a small exchange. Activities were set up for the passengers and children. In the lounge area there might be card games, other games, movies, dances, and a casino night with play money. Those were a few of the activities.

The day of departure, we assisted the doctor, down on the dock. in receiving passengers, not the troops, but the retired people and the children. The active-duty officers came through us on the dock. We reviewed immunization records, medical information forms, history forms. We also observed if they had any health problems we might need to deal with once they got aboard. We gave them information right away where they should come to see us. Later on, we had a briefing for all the passengers.

The troops came on board at a different level of the ship. The chief hospital corpsman and the hospital corpsmen took care of them. I didn't have anything to do with the troops. Periodically, we would have an active-duty doctor or nurse traveling on the ship. We always kept an eye open for any medically trained passengers in case we had difficulties and needed help.

The USNS ships, at one time, had been Army transportation ships that were used during the war periods in the Pacific. The Army would take wounded people from land to the nearest hospital. They were not hospital ships at that time. We did not allow any women on board who were over six months pregnant. Although we could do a delivery, the doctors and I certainly did not want to be involved with it. I had been involved with deliveries in the emergency room at Detroit Receiving, where you just had your OB Pack, the person on a gurney, and you and the doctor caught the baby.

Leaving Oakland, California, going under the Golden Gate Bridge, the sea was pretty rough. That first day out we would usually have man overboard drills. The people would get to their cabins. Then, we would go under the bridge. We would have people with motion sickness, vomiting, headaches, etc. The first few days the medical department would be the busiest. The corpswaves and I would take care of women and children. We would go to their staterooms and provide Dramamine, Bonamine, Compazine or whatever our standing orders were. We would also make rounds and provide crackers, oranges and apples.

The stewards were really good about letting us know, especially me and the corpswaves, if any of the little children or ladies were very seasick and wouldn't come out of their cabin. I would make rounds well before breakfast time, while they were still in their bunks, in order to give them medication and encourage them to get up, get out of the cabin and get into the dining room to eat. During my time, we only had one lady we had to admit to the hospital to give IVs because she was so dehydrated from the motion sickness.

After the first couple of busy days, we would have things like upper respiratory infections and minor injuries. One time, going into Japan, we ran into quite a storm. The ship was listing and pitching. I made rounds to people in the lounge who were afraid to go to their cabins. I gave out medication. Then, I went to my cabin and put on blue jeans, tennis shoes, a sweat shirt and my life jacket and went to sleep on my bunk. The corpsmen never disturbed me. They did have some casualties come down to the hospital. They had the corpswaves come down and help. The doctor would treat minor injuries from falling or banging an arm or a leg. With the listing and pitching, to try and be in full uniform just wouldn't work.

The medical staff, the doctors and I were usually out on deck the day of departure, standing by as the passengers were going down the gangplank, just in case there were any problems with anyone. That pretty much winds up MSTS. It was quite an experience. I never regretted it.

From 1964 to 1965 I was at Oakland Naval Hospital for 11 months. I was in charge of the orthopedic ward. We had amputees, but they were usually casualties that were young men thrown out of a pickup truck or an accident type thing. It was a fairly active orthopedic section. I wasn't in the main hospital, but down in the wooden type buildings, the ramps. It was interesting because two wards might be connected, with utility rooms in between. You could walk from one ward right over to the other ward. It was interesting how the fellows would help take care of each other, or they would go on liberty together.

I had decided to get out of the service. My parents were elderly with increasing health problems. Our family doctor had passed away and they didn't have a doctor. I got out of the service for a year with the idea that I would come back. I was also going to work on my master's. I started to work and help with my parents, so I didn't go back to the university. I did go back in the service in a year.

I was out of the service from 1965 to 1966. I was back in Detroit living in the family house. I stayed in the non-pay reserve unit and did correspondence courses. When I came back on active duty in 1966, I was very fortunate. I was back for about a year and was picked up for lieutenant commander. I also had my same base pay date because I had done reserve duty. My parents' health did deteriorate, but they were under a doctor's care and things looked better by then.

When I came back, I got orders to Philadelphia Naval Hospital. The duty at Philadelphia was a lot of casualties and amputees. I was working the surgical ward with appendectomies and hand surgery. I did have one night that I was covering the ramps, where we had several wards with amputes. It was so emotional to walk on a ward with forty beds and everyone was an amputee of one kind or another. We did have a few retired people with our active-duty people also.

One night I got called at two or three in the morning. The corpsman said they wanted me to come because the doctor wanted a can of beer. I didn't understand that. He said, "Well, it's locked up in the refrigerator, Ma'am." When I got there, the doctor was in the treatment room cutting off the cast of a patient who had just come to the ward within the last hours. I asked the corpsman if that was usual, if he would come in the middle of the night to cut a cast off and order a can of beer for someone. The corpsman said "yes." This doctor felt so strongly that as soon as the patients got on the ward, he was going to get those horrible-smelling casts off and the wounds cleaned up. The men had been in those casts for hours or days. It was something that was so genuinely caring of that doctor. I learned that those orthopedic doctors would give the very best care to these men that were coming back.

The patients helped each other so much. I would walk on the ward at 4:35 in the morning and some of them would be up and getting cleaned up. Then, they would help their buddy. They encouraged each other as they were getting their prostheses. I had seen some very drastic and horrible things while working at the emergency room at Detroit Receiving, but this was something again. Such injuries of young bodies, but such a spirit of hope and help extended to each other. It just made my job easier at times. It changed our lives.

I was at Philadelphia for a year when I got a call from my chief nurse. She said the director of the Navy Nurse Corps had called. They had a position at Newport, Rhode Island, at the Women Officers' School. I hadn't been lieutenant commander very long. Women's Officers' School was my fifth duty station. It was set up to indoctrinate and instruct in subjects such as the Navy department, how the medical department fits into the overall Navy department, military leadership involving the chain of command, ranks, rates, courtesies and naval history. We also received a brief coverage of different ships, planes, weapons, and involvement with marching and inspections. The officers were supplied and fitted with their uniforms. We had several classes on grooming, swimming. There were room inspections of the quarters where the nurses and officers were living and watches and day activities. There was one hour where we dealt with duty assignments, naval hospitals and other type duties a nurse might be assigned. If everything worked okay after the first week, we might have weekend liberty. All of this was to prepare the officer for what they would face in the military hospital or duty station.

I started out as staff advisory for a number of months. Then, the senior nurse at Newport, got orders to Da Nang. I was fleeted up to be the senior nurse and assistant officer in charge. We had women line officers and physical therapy officers there, as well as the nurse corps.

In those years, 1967 to 1969, we got large summer classes there, 100 to 150 people. The time there was cut down to five weeks. Every month and a half we were looking at a new class coming through. We got a small break between classes, maybe a week off. For years afterwards, I may see a nurse, or even now at the association meetings, a nurse will say, "Oh, I went through an officers' school when you were there." They remember me, but I can't remember them. I remember some who were no longer nursing, but they may be a doctor or they finished nursing and at a much higher rank than I was.

I asked for hospital shipboard duty. Even though I had previous shipboard duty, I was given this duty. From December 1969 to December 1970, I was assigned to the hospital ship USS *Repose* for three months and the USS *Sanctuary* for nine months. The *Repose* was called the Angel of the Orient. The ship had served in that area several times during the Korean War and in the Philippines. It was in service already in the forties. It was revamped and modernized in 1965 and came to Vietnam in 1966. Its purpose was to provide offshore medical support to the United States and allied military forces in the number one corps tactical zone of the Republic of Vietnam.

Vietnam was divided into three sections. The ship was offshore from Chu Lai, Thu Bai, Da Nang and Dang Ha. This ship would usually anchor one to two miles offshore in the daytime and receive wounded or ill soldiers, sailors or Marines. They would receive them by helicopter or boat. At night the ship would steam very slowly three to five knots offshore. The ship was painted completely white with red crosses. At night the ship was completely illuminated with white. It was always kept that way. Helicopters coming in could land on the helicopter deck on the stern.

The *Repose* and the *Sanctuary* were very similar. Each was fully equipped as a hospital. It was completely air conditioned. It had 506 hospital beds but could expand to 720 beds. There were four operating rooms. We had a staff of 24 medical, three dental, seven medical services corps, 29 nurse corps and 19 line and supply officers, two chaplains, 246 hospital corpsmen, seven dental techs, 290 ship's crew and two female American Red Cross workers.

Nurses were assigned to different wards. The SOQ (senior officer quarters) had 34 beds. Three medical wards held 48, 34, and 82 patients respectfully. Sometimes there would be a passageway in between these wards. It was considered all one ward. Orthopedics had 33 beds, ENT 24, urology 24, general and thoracic surgery 63, ICU 18, plastic and neurosurgery 42 and the international Vietnamese ward 34 beds plus 2 cribs. There was the recovery room and four operating rooms.

The nurses were assigned to a specific area and pretty much stayed in that area. Some of us had supervision on PM's and nights. If we weren't on duty, we had liberty. We could be in the nurses' quarters in civilian clothes, the sun deck for sun bathing or another deck where they played basketball. Once out of quarters, we had to be in uniform to go to our meals. The nurses assigned to the ship were senior lieutenant JGs, lieutenants, or lieutenant commanders. The JGs had at least one complete two-year hospital tour behind them. I think this was very important because this really was a different isolated type of duty. The ship would, many times, be up and down the coast. We always would have one ship that would be on station. The ship would be there anywhere from 70 to 90 days. Then, we would go to Subic Bay, Philippines, for ship maintenance and supply replenishment. If we had liberty in the Philippines, we would be there for recreation. If we weren't on duty, we could take advantage of walking on the ground and eating greener, which I really appreciated.

We received patients by small boat or helicopter. There was a helipad on the stern of the ship. As soon as the patients arrived, they would go through triage. Medical patients went directly to their ward. Some patients went directly to the operating or recovery room waiting to go into the OR. After treatment, some of the men went back to their duty station ashore. Many of them were medevacked by helicopter off the ship and flown to Clark Air Force Base in the Philippines. Some went to the naval hospital in Guam or Yokosuka, Japan, and then stateside to the various hospitals. The patients would be on the stretcher. Some had complete pajamas and bathrobes. Some just had an exposed chest, but they always had a sheet over them and strapped to the gurney. They also had an information tag and medication if necessary. On the helicopter, they were properly identified and protected from the weather. From the helicopter to the plane, the Air Force nurses would have all the information they needed. For many of them, it was a long trip home. Many of them did get home, which was the wonderful thing about having the hospital ship right there close to where the battles were going on.

The patients would come from the jungle in their fatigues and boots. These would all be stripped off. If they went back to duty with their units, a liaison from their troops, Army, Navy or Marine would see that they were properly uniformed. Also, valuables were taken, documented in the ward, locked up and properly handled until they were able to leave.

On the *Repose*, I was in charge of ICU for three months. I am not a certified ICU nurse. I did not have as much experience in ICU as some other nurses. But I had all this general nursing experience. I had experience in surgical wards and emergency room and was the proper rank. That was to be my third Christmas at sea. When I was at MSTS, I was at sea for two Christmases. I was assigned to be on the *Repose* on 15 December. For women in the service, I think that was a little unusual. I figured I had traveled at least 140 nautical miles at sea. I don't know if any other Navy nurse can claim that record.

I didn't become a Shellback like some of the other Shellbacks. I did go through an initiation on MSTS. After it was done, I went to my cabin, took off the blue jeans, tennis shoes, undergarments and sweatshirt and threw them out the porthole.

In March 1970, the war seemed to be changing. The fierceness and activity were deescalating. It was decided that the *Repose* was going to be called back to the States. Only the *Sanctuary* would stay on station. There were times when the two hospital ships would rendezvous for part of a day in different places along the coast. We would visit each other's ship, see friends or have sports type activities. This happened several times. On March 13, when it was decided the *Repose* was going to be recalled back to the States, we met. We again had some sports functions and a cookout.

On 14 March we had a departure ceremony. It was a formal program with music and words by the chaplain and CO. After the ceremony was over, the guests were invited to the sun deck for refreshments and a ceremony. We said goodbye to the *Sanctuary*. As we were leaving, the Home Going Pendant was attached and raised. This was a pendant that was a long streamer type flag and rose with helium balloons. It was right next to the ship's American flag. It flew over the helicopter deck and stern of the ship. This flew until we were out of sight of the *Sanctuary*. Later on, the crew received a small cutting of the pendant.

We had 16 nurses that flew back to the *Sanctuary* to finish our year.

In my case, it was nine months. When we left the *Repose*, we did have a few patients that were too ill to medevac off the ship. They were in ICU. The ship steamed on to Subic Bay. It also made port in Hong Kong, Kobe, Japan, and Yokosuka. We flew from Yokosuka back to Vietnam and choppered back to the *Sanctuary*. In each port we had liberty. We had four days of liberty in Hong Kong. We stood some duty. I had two days of duty because we had these ill patients in the ICU. The chief nurse and several other nurses stayed with the *Repose* and came home with it because these patients were there too.

When I got on the *Sanctuary*, another nurse was in charge of the ICU. They put us as co-charge of the ICU. The last couple of months I took charge of two medical wards. That was good experience for me because I had primarily worked surgical wards all the time. One day we had already admitted 19 patients. We received and admitted our young men right from the jungle. The helicopter would bring them to the ship. It was announced that so many ambulatory patients were coming. They came to the passageway of the ship by the ward. The corpsmen would have them sit down. Then, they were taken to the shower area. They'd have a plastic bag with a bathrobe, pajamas and cloth slippers inside. They would also be given a ditty bag with toothpaste, toothbrush, a razor, and soap. They would get into the shower area, get out of their uniform, put it in a plastic bag and give that to the corpsmen. They would then shower and come out the other way and be assigned a bed. Vital signs would be taken. Some would be helped if needed. I had just gotten back to my room, taken off my uniform and laid on my bunk in my slip. I was going to rest before going to dinner when they announced over the loud speaker there were 30 ambulatory patients. I got up, got dressed and went to help the afternoon shift. You just got up and helped.

The bunks were at least two-tiered, some three. The sicker patients or those with IVs were put in the lower bunks. The ICU was very intense and the injuries very drastic. We had two striker beds and one circle-electric bed. We also might have a Vietnamese baby or child in the crib in the ICU unit. There were four or five corpsmen on duty. You had the senior nurse and one or two other nurses most of the time. It was pretty intense. The doctors were wonderful though. They would be close by and stay close.

Besides having our normal duties, we would also have recovery room duty. In recovery room, we received patients from triage before they went in and after they came out of the operating room. When we were off shore from Da Nang and not up the line, we might have enemy frogmen swimming around the ship. Our crew would drop hand grenades over the side. One time, I was in the recovery room below the water level. They had dropped a grenade over the side and the percussion knocked stuff off the bulkhead. At one point the ship would just anchor and stay off the shoreline of Da Nang. When they were suspecting frogmen, we were moving all the time. We couldn't just anchor and stay there.

In December 1970, my year in Vietnam was over. I flew home on the Freedom Bird. I was glad to come home. When I got on the ship, I heard some of the nurses and doctors talking about the Freedom Bird. I didn't know what they were talking about. They were talking about American Airlines, which brought us to Vietnam and also took us home. The Freedom Bird was when people had orders to come back to the States. That last month I didn't want to get off the ship because I didn't want anything to happen to me, although, if I got injured, I would be sent home. A strange feeling comes over you because you are a part of that crew and a part of that ship. There is such a need that you are not sure about how you're going to be when you get home.

I left with a nurse and a doctor who had come to Vietnam with me. The nurse invited me to stay in California overnight with her family. She and her sister had arranged for our hair to be done at a beauty shop the next day. After a day and a night, I flew back home to Detroit to my parents' home. I didn't feel really strange or anything when I was home. No one gave me any trouble about coming home in Detroit.

I went on to Bremerton Naval Hospital from 1971 to 1974. I think that was a good duty station because there were a small number of nurses. The hospital wasn't overly active. I felt it was a time for readjustment. It was an easy pace. I worked the ER and CSR. I went in as an experienced nurse, but I learned an awful lot. I did supervision when it was my turn. I did this for a year and a half. Then, I went up to the office for clinical detailing. The nurses were really assigned by the assistant chief nurse. I mainly assigned the corpsmen, which I liked very much. The nurses were a close group. The civilian nurses that worked in the clinic and on some of the wards were very friendly. It was a good time for me at Bremerton.

I had senior nurses who were mentors to me. I was treating my patients as I would want to be treated. I tried to treat them as if they were my family. These young men wanted to learn and do so much. When I was supervising, I loved going through the nursery and seeing a corpsman the size of a football player gently handling these little babies. They are just wonderful memories.

I left Bremerton in 1974. I left with a hardship move because my parents were elderly and had some medical problems. Before I was granted the hardship move, my mother passed away. The Navy still honored my hardship request and I was moved to Great Lakes. My father lived another 15 months, which was great. I could drive home from Great Lakes to Detroit in six or seven hours. I had that time with him. I was very thankful to the Navy for granting me that.

At Great Lakes, I started as a clinical detail officer, taking care of the corpsmen and nurses. That was quite a challenge. Great Lakes was more active and larger than Bremerton, where I was doing corpsmen detail. From 1978 to 1982, I moved to Naval Hospital, Portsmouth, Virginia. I covered the dependent wards. Several times, for a month or so at a time, I covered the nursing office, which is very rewarding. I felt I had a very rewarding and wonderful career in the Navy. It was actually half of my adult life.

I retired out of Portsmouth in 1982 and went back to Detroit. I stayed in Virginia for a year as a transition time. I felt that was a very wise move on my part. I was able to associate with the nurses, but I didn't have to punch a clock. It gave me time to start my adjustment to civilian life. I decided that I would probably go back to Michigan. What family I had was still in Michigan.

I've been very thankful and proud to serve. I've been thankful for all the encouragement, guidance and respect that was given to me at my different duty stations by senior nurses, line officers, medical service corps officers, my peers and corps staff. Many times, we forget that we are giving to the patient but the patient is giving back to us more than we realize—more hope, love and faith in us than we realize. I've felt that a number of times with patients, whether they were military or civilians. Those friendships that we've made over the years were friendships at the duty stations and some are still with me today. All those friendships and people I've had contact with along the way I feel sometimes it influenced me and I hope that I have influenced them as well.

Irma Klaetke passed away on 31 October 2021. This account is being included in this book with the consent of Irma's brother, George H. Klaetke.

Helen Bergin Kranz

Helen was planted in the Philippines during the Vietnam War, a little distant from the fighting. She bloomed there, having wonderful experiences caring for casualties from Vietnam and gaining experience that impacted the rest of her life.

I WAS BORN AND RAISED in Waltham, Massachusetts. I am the fourth oldest of ten kids. We all went to college because my parents told us we didn't have a choice. My father wanted me to go to a state BSN program in Massachusetts. I applied to nursing schools because I liked biology. I did not get into the state's BSN school, but I did get accepted into the three diploma programs to which I applied. I went to St. Elizabeth's Hospital School of Nursing in Boston. I graduated from high school in 1967, started at St. Elizabeth's in September 1967, graduated in June 1970. I completed my BSN at the University of New Hampshire in 1988 using the GI bill.

It has been over 52 years, June 1969, since I was commissioned an ensign in the U.S. Navy Nurse Corps in Boston, Massachusetts, by my brother, a recruiter lieutenant in the U.S. Navy waiting to get into medical school in Denver, Colorado. Those early years were so impactful. They went by so fast. I was just going along and accepting the wonderful experiences that were happening to me.

My senior year in nursing school I was getting a monthly check that paid my tuition. I paid my parents back for the first two years of nursing school. I think my monthly check was $125. It went a long way back then. Nursing school tuition was $800 a year.

I went to Newport, Rhode Island, at the end of June 1970 for the officer indoctrination program. There were 125 people in my class. It was considered a very large class. We were there for about a month. I had already received orders to go to Camp LeJeune, North Carolina. I had no idea where it was. I had to look it up on a map. My mother made it out to be such a great adventure that I would see the world. Both of my parents were so happy for me. My father was a World War II veteran, serving 26 years in the United States Air Force Reserve.

I got to Camp Lejeune in August 1970. I started working on the dependents' floor because when I took my RN boards, I did not pass the medical part. The boards were two days of testing, handwritten, with six parts: surgical, OB, medical, psych, geriatrics and pediatrics. When I didn't pass, I did not have an RN license. I was told I couldn't carry the keys to the narcotics locker. I was assigned to a dependents' floor because there were civilian nurses there who carried keys and were in charge. I had to fly back to Boston to retake the certification test in September. I found out a week later that I had passed.

I continued to work dependents' for about six months. Then, I was transferred to the surgical ICU. We all lived in the nurses' quarters at Camp Lejeune. I worked in the surgical ICU where I learned so much. We treated Vietnam War casualties that, in some cases, were less than a few days from the battlefield. The wards were packed with fifty or more patients who were sick and traumatized. I spent at least a year in ICU. We worked very hard and went home exhausted after every shift. The patients were either local from training accidents or complicated cases from the battlefield.

While I was there, we had 12 cases of meningitis. It was from living in close quarters in wet tents at Camp Geiger. They were all 18 to 20–year-old Marines. A couple of them died. I was horrified that that could happen. The average age of our patients was 20 years old. Occasionally we would get a retired Marine in with a heart attack. We had a CCU next to us that could expand into a 24 bed ICU. But there had never been more than 15 patients in there. We did have pediatric patients occasionally who would be pretty sick.

Back then, the Marines would come back from Vietnam and either go to Camp Lejeune or Bethesda on the East Coast or Camp Pendleton on the West Coast. They would try to get them as close to the state where they were from. They were really sick Marines because these were all battle injuries. There were a lot of amputations and surgical patients with grenade or machine gun injuries.

I met my husband at the officers' club. He was hurting because he had just returned from Vietnam about six months earlier. I think I understood where he was coming from because every now and then he would talk a little about what he had been through. When I found out he had a bronze star and a purple heart, I knew he had seen a lot of action.

We began dating. One time, we went to the movies. He met this sergeant that he had known when he was in-country. The guy came up and hugged him. They talked for a few minutes and said they would get together. They were so happy to see each other because each of them thought the other had been killed. Each of them had rotated out of Vietnam at different times. The Marines would stay for twelve months, but they all came home at different times. They would be with a group for three months. Then, they would never see each other again. One of the first things officers did when they got in-country would be to throw away their bars. The insignia would reflect the sun and give away their rank. All the men had nicknames. The nicknames would make it so they never called each other by rank. Officers were the first to be targeted by the enemy. He was with the 3rd Marine Division, 9th Marine 3/9 north of Da Nang, actually into North Vietnam.

After being at Camp Lejeune for nine months, he got orders to Guantanamo Bay, Cuba (Gitmo). I would get a letter through the "God mail" system. The wife of the USMC senior officer in Gitmo lived on base. She would put a shoebox out in her garage. You could drive down a back alley to get to her garage. When the mail would come in from Gitmo to Cherry Point, she would get all the mail and put all the letters in the shoebox. Even though we weren't married, my husband got permission to write me. I could go once or twice a week to the shoebox and get the letters. I would get about two letters a week. We couldn't get them through the regular mail because Gitmo was out of country. I would drop my letters off to the shoebox to get my letters down to my boyfriend. When he came back to Camp Lejeune, we continued to date. We got engaged in the summer of 1971. We were married the following April 15, 1972.

We were both going to get out of the military. We went to a couple of job fairs. He couldn't really find a job. He decided to stay in the Marine Corps. He got orders to Subic Bay in the Philippines. I was going to get out of the Navy when I had fulfilled my obligation in June 1972. My husband wanted me to get out and come over to the Philippines as a civilian wife. My brother said that when he was in Vietnam, he went to the Philippines on R&R. He said that there was an agreement signed for the U.S. to have a base in the Philippines. The civilian jobs had to be filled by Philippine citizens and not civilian Americans. My father thought I should try staying in the Navy and seeing if I could go over as a Navy nurse. The Navy said I could get orders to Subic. There were only 12 Navy nurses stationed at Subic Naval Hospital. The only nurse opening was for the OR nurse. I wasn't qualified. The chief nurse at Camp Lejeune had me go through an OR rotation because I had an OR rotation in nursing school. My husband left for the Philippines in June 1972. I was able to get orders and left in July.

My 14 months in Subic are like they happened yesterday, not fifty years ago. I remember that my mother dropped me off at Logan Airport in Boston in August 1972. My Mom told me to think of my assignment as a wonderful adventure to see new places and meet new people as she kissed and hugged me goodbye at the airport. I was very excited to go to a new country. I was really looking forward to seeing my husband again and setting up our new household on base. I didn't think much about the patients I would be treating because I thought I had seen everything at Camp Lejeune in the ICU. I arrived in the Philippines in August 1972, after a very long flight from Travis Air Force Base in California via Alaska. I was a 21-year-old Navy nurse with two years of nursing experience under my belt in med surg and ICU nursing from Camp LeJeune Naval Hospital.

My husband met me at Clark Air Force Base. He said, "I have good news and bad news. The good is that we can stay here overnight and get a helicopter ride back to Subic tomorrow instead of driving." It was only sixty miles, but it took hours and hours because it was over a dirt road. "The bad news is that I moved into base housing (a townhouse situation with two bedrooms and bath upstairs and living, dining, porch and kitchen downstairs) two days ago. I was broken into. They stole everything." The townhouse was located on the perimeter of the base a couple of miles from the hospital and with a beautiful view of the bay. The intruders cut through the barbed wire and broke into our townhouse. They stole a clock and all the wedding gifts I had shipped over with my husband's shipment. He was asleep upstairs when this happened. They went all the way upstairs, into our bedroom and stole his watch and ID card. The watch and USMC ID card was on the black market the next day. They stole his money and came downstairs into the kitchen. He had bought a couple of steaks and some eggs. They left him one steak and one egg. That was because they say that they are Christian and take care of each other. They didn't wake him, stab him, or kill him. They left him something to eat, but they took everything else. On the way out the back door, they stabbed the guard. He was at the naval hospital when we arrived.

When I got there, I found out about all this. My husband had taken on the job of being the coach for the football team to keep himself busy until I got there. That was a big deal because they played each base all over the Pacific. All these admirals and generals were playing each other. It was a like a military football league. My husband was the linebacker coach.

We took the chopper ride back to base. The chopper pilot took me over the hospital so I could see it. On the way, we went over the Marine

Amphibious Unit (MAU), a Marine training camp before the Marines went to Vietnam. My husband's job at Cubie Point was the executive officer of Separate Guard Company. They are responsible for guarding the main magazine. The magazine was where all the ammunition was stored for the ships that would come into port rotating to and from Vietnam. The magazine was in the far north corner of the base. We lived on the far south corner of the base. Cubie Point was way up on a mountain.

The next day my husband had to go with the football team. I walked through the hospital and nobody knew who I was. There were four wards, an OR and an ER. I wondered what I was going to do for a week. I went into the chief nurse's office, introduced myself and I checked in a week early. They said, "We didn't expect you for another week." I said, "I know, but I'm here." I told the chief nurse to put me on nights or PMs. She put me on PMs. Checking into the Subic Bay Naval Hospital, I was assigned to a med/surg floor with 65 patients. The head nurse was an experienced nurse who had a great command of the staff and the floor. When she saw I had ICU experience, she informed me when we had critical patients I would be involved.

I remember one patient who was transferred in from one of the hospital ships that came into the harbor. He was on a ventilator and too sick to transport to the U.S. Back in those days, patients on a ventilator were not transferred back to the U.S. We made a corner of the open bay Ward B, near the nurses' desk, his curtained area. A corpsman and Navy nurse were assigned to him for every shift. It was touch and go for a while. After a week, he was weaned off the ventilator over a few days. Eventually, he was sent to Camp Pendleton Naval Hospital, when stable enough to move. He had many wounds and lots of drains and IVs. He never regained consciousness while under our care, but we were thrilled that he could finally breathe on his own. I always wondered what happened to him after he left our little 100 bed hospital.

At Subic, the patients were very sick on the Medical Surgical Floor where I was assigned. I also had to take operating room call, which did scare me since my OR experience had only been in nursing school and the review I received at Camp Lejeune before I transferred to Subic. There was a horrific motorcycle accident on base one night. I was on call for the operating room duty. One service member had been killed and the other had traumatic head wounds and a fractured pelvis. I was called in, as was the backup nurse. There were two of us and a few MDs. I learned a lot that night and the patient made it to recovery. The Marine that was killed was on his R&R from Vietnam. He wasn't killed in Vietnam, but was killed in a sad motorcycle accident. This could be an example of the irony in life.

Subic Bay Naval Hospital had 13 Navy nurses and many Filipino RN's. There were also Philippine medical students from Manila that rotated through various specialties. The Navy nurses would teach the Philippine med students how to draw blood and start IVs. The patients never really knew who was who. The Philippine students were very eager to learn and grateful for the opportunities provided at the naval hospital.

All the nurses, except me, lived in the nurses' quarters across the street from the hospital. I stayed there, as well, when I had the duty. They each had a nice room and bathroom. They had a wonderful cook. She would cook three meals a day. When I was working, I could go over and have lunch there. The nurses' quarters were a happy place. We went to many a pig roast and barbecue up there. There was one other married nurse. Her husband was Air Force retired, so she lived off base.

We were actually in Manila at the end of September 1972, when Marcos declared martial law. We were at the Philippine-American officers' club, right by the embassy, having dinner. The waiter came to our table and told us we had to go back to our hotel right away for safety because martial law was being declared. There weren't any cabs, so we had to walk a couple of blocks. We were staying at the Hyatt. They had all their shades down and told us to stay away from the windows. All night long we heard these jeepneys going up and down. We heard gunfire. The next day they took us to the embassy and told us we had to go back to Subic. They evacuated us. Martial law was in effect the rest of the time we were there.

I was supposed to stay 15 months, but was expecting our first son. Back then you could not stay in the military once you were pregnant. My husband was due to rotate back in September. In July, I was four months pregnant, seeing the doctor at the naval hospital and doing great. I worked a very busy surgical floor, a lot of medevacs in and out. I was told I couldn't work with the sailors or Marines. I asked the chief nurse why and was told it was because I couldn't be near any military being pregnant. I was assigned to the pediatric immunization clinic. The chief nurse was very old fashioned. I was allowed to wear a white pant suit. It looked the same as a Navy uniform. I got to wear my military pant suit uniforms with military insignia. My other uniforms didn't fit me. They didn't have maternity Navy uniforms at the time. I'd always wear civilian clothes when everyone else would be wearing their uniforms for inspection. I wouldn't have to go to the inspections.

That was the month that an Air Force flight nurse took it all the way to the Supreme Court in a case against pregnant women getting kicked out of the military. The Supreme Court ruled in her favor. I was told I could still stay in the Navy. When my husband rotated back to the States, I was allowed to go with him. They cut my tour short. We were assigned to Camp Pendleton.

I had the baby in November and left active-duty status. I wanted to get into the reserves. A young lieutenant MSC told me to stay home and take care of my family. There was really no place in the Navy for women who had children. I remember saying, "Well, men have children and they stay in the Navy." He said, "It doesn't matter. There are no billets." I said, "I'm not going to give up. I want to get back in the Navy, in the reserves." He said, "There is no place for you in the Navy." I kept calling and calling him, driving him crazy. He finally said, "Okay, you can drill, but you won't get paid for it." I said, "That doesn't seem fair." He said, "Take it or leave it." So, I took it.

I drilled at Camp Pendleton in the clinic with a wonderful lieutenant commander. She'd say, "Can you come in for four hours? We'll count it as a drill." One drill equaled four hours. I'd get a babysitter and go in. I found out there were 24 paid drills. In other words, you drill 48 but you only get paid for 24. So, I started calling down to San Diego saying I wanted one of those billets. I said, "I've been drilling for free for maybe six months or more." They got me into a program with 48 drills, but I only got paid for 24. It worked out great. I was thrilled to get a paid billet.

I got pregnant with my second son and continued to drill. They allowed me to do two weeks active duty with pay. I would go back to Camp Pendleton again and work in the same clinic. Whatever that nurse wanted me to do, I'd do. Sometimes it was the surgical clinic, sometimes OB or peds. It was very important to me to stay in the Navy.

I also had a civilian job working at San Clemente General Hospital one day a week. It was right across from Route 5, where President Nixon was living. I worked in an ICU that had eight beds. It was pretty busy. Most of the patients were quite old. I was used to the younger patients in the military. I continued to drill at Camp Pendleton. My husband had to go to Okinawa. At first, they said I could go. Then, it was going to be an unaccompanied tour. If accompanied, it's two years. Unaccompanied, it was a year. We had our second son in September 1975. I ended up moving home to live with my family. He went to Okinawa. We sold our house in California.

I was able to hook up to another 24-pay unit at South Weymouth Naval Air Station in South Weymouth, Massachusetts. Then halfway through the year, I got full pay. This was also a clinic situation. I didn't work as a civilian nurse. I couldn't because my mother was working and all my sisters were either going to school or working. I had the two boys and would drill on my Navy weekends.

When my husband got back, we were stationed in Memphis, Tennessee. He was going to be the I&I instructor inspector at Jackson Avenue USMC Reserve Center in Memphis. We were there from 1976 to 1981. I had two more children at Millington Naval Base. I got a 48-pay drill there. I drilled down on Avery Street Naval Reserve Center and did my active duty at Millington Naval Base. That was a training command. Now, Millington is a personnel command where all the records are kept and where promotion boards are held.

My husband got out of the Marine Corps. We moved up to New Hampshire. I've been here for 41 years. I transferred into the Navy reserve. I was attached to Lawrence, Massachusetts, for nine years. I was the training officer, XO, then, the OIC. The last three years at the Lawrence Reserve Center, I was the CO of the Bethesda unit, with active duty at Bethesda, Maryland. I became the CO of a unit in Portsmouth, New Hampshire. It was only about a half hour from where I lived. I was stationed out of Manchester. I was also the REDCOM nurse for a couple of years down in Newport, Rhode Island.

Sometimes I'd be the only woman commanding officer in the whole reserve center. In Lawrence, Massachusetts, I'd go in during the week to turn in my reports. The petty officers that were stationed there were right off the ships and some were pretty vulgar. They had pinups and *Playboy* calendars in the training office. I was offended by it. The CO was a lot younger than me. I went in and told him that I didn't think that was appropriate. He said, essentially, he didn't care what I thought. I told a captain in Washington headquarters. She said I had rights and I needed to take it to the REDCOM (Readiness Command in Newport, Rhode Island). They were all sailors off ships stationed as REDCOM as well. They couldn't have cared less what I thought. Finally, we resolved that the sailors would take the calendars down when reservists were around and put them back up as soon as we'd leave. This was before the Tailhook Incident happened. I remember that to this day how I thought it was disgusting. The female reservists all felt the Navy had to change. I am happy to say that by the time I retired attitudes were changing.

I retired on October 10, 1999, at the USS *Constitution* in Boston, Massachusetts, as a Captain, Nurse Corps, U.S. Navy, after 30 years of honorable service. The Navy was the best experience I have ever had. I am proud to have served.

All these years later, I am being asked about my choice to join the military. Going in the Navy was the smartest thing I ever did for myself. First of all, I was on a scholarship that paid for my three-year nursing school. By accepting a nursing scholarship, I made my career a reality. This career in the military took me all over the world. I met people I never would have met. I saw things I never would have seen. I loved it all.

I grew up fast. At the age of 20, I was in charge of sick patients at Camp Lejeune Naval Hospital, Jacksonville, North Carolina. I could not vote or even get a loan to buy a car without a co-signer back in 1970, but I had an ID card that said I was covered under the Geneva Convention if ever captured. I felt so important and so needed, not just as an RN but as a member of the military. My life mattered to many others. I was part of a team and was doing something for my country. It was awesome!

These positive feelings have never left me. My husband and I were a military family. We both loved our time in the military.

My reserve career was challenging, but so rewarding. I learned the language of reserve lingo, such as what is a drill and how are we paid for double time doing four-hour drills. I held some different jobs such as training officer, assistant officer in charge, executive officer and commanding officer. I learned so much about administrative requirements and Navy organization. I did two weeks on active duty every year and even spent two weeks in the desert setting up a field hospital. It was a wild and exciting experience.

These experiences affected my civilian life in so many ways. I was proud to wear the uniform. In the 1970s, when we were told we could not travel in uniform because of anti-military rhetoric in the public, I was so shocked and hurt. This stayed with me forever. People did not care that we were Vietnam era veterans or where we had been stationed or what we did. The attitude of the public was disrespect for veterans.

Years later, when we settled in New Hampshire, I pushed my husband to join the American Legion. This was a very good decision for both of us. We are active members, but the best part was we met veterans who have been stationed where we were, experienced travel and places where we have been. It has helped my husband make wonderful veteran friends, which in turn makes my life better.

In review, the decision to join the Navy was one of, if not the best, decision of my career and life. I have no regrets. I have had a wonderful journey and continue to remember and be proud of what I accomplished.

Susan Stuart Miller

I GRADUATED FROM HIGH SCHOOL in 1962 from Mckinley High School in Canton, Ohio. I went to the University of Cincinnati College of Nursing, a four-year baccalaureate program. It was an excellent nursing school. A significant influence in my life was my mother, who was a nurse. She had gone to a diploma school and encouraged me to go to college. She said, "I don't want you going to a diploma school. I want you to get the benefits of college, too." I had a good time in nursing school and made a lot of good friends that I still see at reunions.

Finances were tight in nursing school because my brother was in dental school. Several of us students heard about the Navy Nurse Corps Candidate Program. We went into Cincinnati to see a Navy recruiter. I signed up in the last part of my sophomore year. It paid my junior and senior year. I owed the Navy three years. I was the first one in the military in my family. I set the precedent. My two brothers followed, my older brother as a dental officer, my younger brother as an Army draftee. During Vietnam there were three of us in the military. The Navy Nurse Corps Candidate Program was a great program. It was the best decision I ever made. It really changed my life.

I went to Officer Candidate School in Newport, Rhode Island. I drove my little Volkswagen there and had it during indoctrination. School was shortened to four weeks because it was 1966 and we were starting to get involved in Vietnam. They needed nurses quickly. My first duty station was Camp Pendleton, California. I gave my VW to my brother in dental school, flew out to California and bought a new car, a Chevy Camaro. It was my first time away from home except for college. I did this all by myself. At the time I didn't realize how scary it was. I didn't think about being homesick or nervous. I just did it. My parents were very supportive and proud of me. My father had tears in his eyes many times because he was so proud of me. My mother was, of course, very proud I was a nurse. To be a Navy nurse was even more impressive. Some of my mother's friends were in the Army Nurse Corps during World War II.

148

I got to Camp Pendleton in October 1966 and served there for a year and a half. I knew very little about clinical nursing on a floor. The corpsmen taught us ensigns a lot about actual bedside procedures, which we hadn't learned in college. Some senior nurses helped to teach us, also. All-in-all, we were good nurses because we knew the process of nursing. We just didn't know a lot of the technical part.

Camp Pendleton was an old, World War II pavilion hospital. It was set up like an H. One wing was the medical side and the other wing surgical. I served on the medical side, which included six or seven wards. During the night shift you would cover all the wards supervising the corpsmen. Sometimes we would drive little carts up and down the ramps because you couldn't get from one end to the other without one. During the day shifts, we would work special wards such as medical, medical ICU, psych, ENT and emergency room. There were quite a few ensigns that came at the same time, so we were all learning together. They became my good friends and some of them are still my friends today.

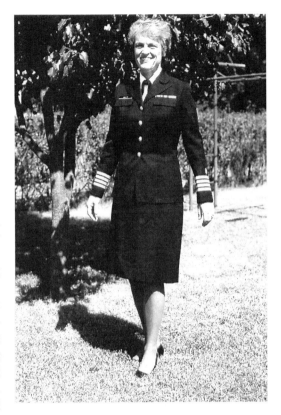

Susan Stuart Miller (taken 1985 in Salisbury, Maryland). Susan had just been commissioned captain. Photo by permission.

Mostly, my experience at Camp Pendleton was just being very naïve, young and needing to learn a lot. I did learn a lot and had a good time living by myself for the first time in an apartment. I learned how to be on my own and pay my own bills. That was the biggest part of Camp Pendleton.

I got orders to Naval Hospital Guam in March 1968. Vietnam was ramping up. Lots of nurses were sent overseas. Several of us from Camp

Pendleton got sent to Guam together, so I did have a few friends with me. I actually asked for overseas, but I don't think Guam was on my list. It turned out to be the greatest experience of my life to work on Guam during the Vietnam War. We did so much work and helped so many patients. We just were a big part of that war.

The hundred bed hospital went to over seven hundred beds within a month or two. They were bringing in nurses and corpsmen. The main hospital was at Agana. Then, they opened up Asan, a hospital annex. This is how they ramped it up to over seven hundred. Asan was a World War II facility reopened for the Vietnam War. It was right after the Tet Offensive. We were getting air-evac patients five times a week, right from Vietnam. We had a triage ward. The patients were triaged, cleaned up and fed and sent to their respective wards for care the next day. It seemed like we would fill the whole ward, about fifty or sixty patients, at one time. We had special triage nurses that worked on that ward. The rest of us worked on other wards and pulled extra duty there. We worked a lot, not only our own shifts, but a lot of extra duty shifts.

The island of Guam is about five by twelve miles. There really was nowhere else to go. I ended up playing golf a lot. There were three golf courses on the island. If I wasn't working, sleeping or partying, I was golfing. Being so active was good because it gave me an outlet for the anxiety created from taking care of all these very sick patients. I actually did have some PTSD. Twenty years later I went to a vet center for counseling. It took twenty years to be able to come out and say I needed some help to deal with my emotions from the war.

The friends I made in Guam are the friends I get together with every two years. I call them "my Guamies." These are doctors, nurses, corpsmen and patients from Guam, basically '68 and '69. They are kind of a core group. We get together to reminisce and remember the good times and how much work we did. There are about fifty of us.

In Guam, we got mostly the shrapnel wounds and amputees. Japan got the burns. We had wards and wards of amputees. We also got a lot of malaria patients that ended up on our medical wards. I worked the intensive care unit most of my time there. It was both surgical and medical. Mostly it ended up being surgical. We would get the severe injuries they couldn't handle on the ward.

It was very hard, stressful work. We couldn't show our emotions, so we just shoved it down and kept shoving it down. You couldn't cry in front of your patients. We had to keep our professionalism. If there were emotions, we just kept shoving them down. I think the nurses have more counseling offered today. We didn't have any counseling or really help of any kind offered to us then. The supervision was definitely to get the

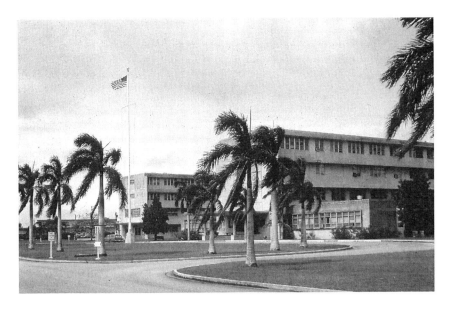

United States Naval Hospital, Guam, taken 1968 by Susan Miller. Photo by permission.

job done and keep your unit clean. There was nothing related to helping our mental status.

I remember the really sick patients and the patients that died on my shift. I remember one Marine who was about eighteen years old. He was pretty much out of it the whole time we had him. He had massive shrapnel injuries. I remember him dying and me being upset about it. One of the other nurses and I started having nightmares after we took care of him. We talked about it and decided to write to his parents, just to let them know he wasn't alone when he died. This was unheard of. You were never supposed to have contact with any of the families of the patients. On our own, we wrote to this Marine's parents, just to let them know that the nurses were with him. We were there holding his hand when he passed. I'll never forget the letter they wrote back. I still have it. They were just so appreciative that he didn't die alone, that he had somebody that loved him and cared about him when he died. We cherish that letter to this day. It was a nurse going out of her comfort zone to do what her gut felt right. I've always believed that you have to do what your gut says is right. Immediately, the nightmares went away. I still definitely listen to my gut feelings.

When I was living in Washington, D.C., my father got sick and was going to go in for some testing in the hospital. He went in for an angiogram. I told the doctors I was working for in Washington I wanted to go home and see him before he went in for these tests. They minimized it and said, "Oh, come on, he's just going in for an angiogram." I said, "No, really. I just have a feeling I want to go home and see him before he goes into the procedure." They let me go, and I flew home. My mother was able to sneak me into the hospital in the evening because it was after visiting hours. I was able to go up and visit my dad and talk to him before he went down for the procedure the next day. They stroked him out during the procedure. He was comatose for three months and then died. That's a story I tell my nursing students all the time. Something in my gut told me I needed to get home and see him before he had that procedure. I tell them to really listen to their own instincts when they have big decisions to make.

I left Guam in 1969. It was in 1987 when I went to a vet center in Baltimore for help. I had never been able to talk about Vietnam. I had never been able to tell anybody, in all those years, about my experiences overseas. I had never discussed anything and couldn't watch movies on Vietnam. Finally, in 1987, I thought maybe something was wrong and I needed to think about this and go get some treatment. At that time the vet center was independent from the VA. I went to the local vet center and had about six months of counseling. I was able to talk about all the stuff I had never been able to talk about. I was able to bring my feelings up and discuss all those feelings I had pushed down all those years.

Fortunately, what I had done during the war was to make audio tapes. I sent tapes home to my parents, in addition to letters. They saved all my tapes. Part of my vet counseling was to listen to my tapes and talk about them each week. It was helpful because it validated my feelings and experience. I could tell by those tapes I had really been dealing with the stress of the war and all the death and dying. Physically, I functioned fine, but emotionally, I just kept shoving it all down. It helped to just talk about the emotions of the war, the sadness and loss of the patients. I had never validated my feelings. That was a big help to know the experience actually was as traumatic as I thought it was.

When I came home from Guam, my parents were very supportive of me and definitely listened. They could tell the war had taken its toll on me. It was hard being a nurse in the war. In 1969, the military was despised in America. When I came home you did not tell people you were in the military. I never wore my uniform, and I got out of the service. Most of the nurses from Guam got out of the service. We were not happy. Good thing for me, I went back into the Navy reserves about six months later. In the long run, that helped me because I stayed close to the military all these years. I think the people that actually got out and did not get back into the reserves may not have had a chance to deal with what they experienced as they were not around other Navy people to discuss it.

My Guamies helped me with my recovery. On Guam, we nurses took care of each other. If one was down, we'd support them. They'd turn around and support us when we were down. It was a very intense close group of nurses that served overseas together. Many times, if one is having trouble, the others will flock to the area to help out. War brings people closer than anything else can bring you.

I needed extra money and so I went back into the reserves in late 1969. I went back to Ohio when I got off active duty and joined the reserves. I liked California, so I moved to San Diego as a civilian at the end of 1969. I continued in the reserves until I retired in 2000. I did a total of 34 years. Three and a half years were active duty. I served as a civilian nurse on the hospital ship SS *Hope* in Brazil in 1973.

I eventually went to Washington, D.C., in 1974. I met a fellow reservist, got married, had two children, but still stayed in the reserves. In the mid– to late '70s it was not as bad to be married in the military as it used to be, as long as you weren't in the same chain of command together. We were both in the reserves. We planned our weekends so he could watch the kids one weekend while I drilled. Then, he would drill and I would watch the kids. Two weekends out of four we had reserve duty. It was good because the kids grew up knowing and liking the military and thinking this was the normal way to do things. Our son served several years in the Army. Our daughter went in the Navy as a naval flight officer for several years. They both grew up with an appreciation of the military, what military people do and the sacrifices we made. We did make a lot of sacrifices through the years to do those two weekends a month plus the two weeks active duty a year.

My husband and I were recalled to active duty for Desert Shield/ Desert Storm. I was stationed at the Bureau of Medicine and Surgery in Washington, D.C., as special assistant to the deputy director Navy Nurse Corps, Reserve Affairs. My husband was called up to Naval Hospital Bethesda as the command master chief for nursing service.

Initially, I was very anxious when Desert Storm started. I was afraid that both of us were going to get sent overseas. Our kids were 12 and 10. We had a backup plan, but we were still anxious. When he got sent to Bethesda and I got sent to Washington, even though we had to make a lot of adaptations, at least we weren't going overseas. We were able to get home most nights. We had to do different shifts so someone could be there in the morning and when the kids came home at night. My neighbors and relatives also helped.

The fleet hospitals were getting activated. Fleet hospitals were made up of people from all over the country. Many reservists wondered why we were bringing onesies and twosies in from all over the country. In reality, they were all part of this major fleet hospital. At the time, it was hard to get a paid billet, so I think a lot of people were saying, "Okay, I'll be part of a fleet hospital even though I have to travel two or three hours to do my drills there." They couldn't imagine that a fleet hospital was going to get activated and sent to war. But there was a plan.

During Desert Storm I learned a lot about the reserve nurses because we were their point of contact in Washington, D.C. We were the ones they'd call if they had a problem. I served five months at BUMED. I left my job in drug addiction permanently. It was time to get a new position. I wanted to get out of nursing. Had I not been called up for active duty, I probably would have gotten out of nursing. However, during my active duty, I was able to rethink everything and that's when I decided to go back to school and become a nurse practitioner. I needed to find a new direction for my nursing career. I already had an MSN in psych/mental health nursing, so I went to George Washington University in Washington, D.C., to get my post master's certificate as an adult nurse practitioner.

As a reservist, I always tried to get the young nurses to look at the big picture, as far as staying in the reserves. Even though it might be rough at the time and they're tired of drilling, I encouraged them to think about the big picture and to get those twenty years in. I've had several nurses come back to me later, as commanders or captains and say, "Thank goodness you told me what you did. I stayed in. Now, I'm going to get my twenty years and my pension."

It is the military experience that teaches organization, priority setting and decision making. If you put two nurses together and one of them is a military nurse, she will outshine the other. She has learned organization, leadership, all those skills. People who have not been in the military cannot understand that way of looking at things. They don't understand why you are so obsessed about organization, setting priorities, saying what you think and doing what you believe in, regardless of what other people think.

I was forever changed by my experience as a Navy nurse during the Vietnam War. I went to Guam in early 1968 as a "young, naïve" nurse who was just starting to develop my nursing skills. I came home from Guam in late 1969 as an "old, weary" nurse, who had been involved in more death and dying than most nurses experience in a lifetime.

Professionally, my skills were highly developed, having worked for a year and a half caring for Marines with amputations, multiple shrapnel wounds, head injuries and all other physical and mental injuries that could have been sustained in a deadly war.

Emotionally I was shut down! I had been pushing my emotions down for a year and a half. Dealing daily with massive injuries to these courageous young men, I could not let my emotions affect my nursing care. I had to keep calm and professional—no crying or getting involved allowed! I had to just keep pushing my emotions down and provide the best care I could. For twenty years after my return from Guam, I kept Vietnam in a hidden place and didn't talk about my Vietnam War experience. I got married, raised a family, and got on with my civilian career. Finally, almost twenty years later, I went to a Vet Center in Baltimore, Maryland, to find out why I felt so numb and closed off about my Vietnam War experience. Only through Vet Center counseling in 1987, did I finally deal with all those sad, depressed emotions that I had buried deep in my soul. I finally processed how overwhelming this experience had been for me. The tapes validated all those feelings that I had buried and reaffirmed my experience dealing with death and dying every day. Now I could finally talk about Vietnam and become involved in healing experiences with my fellow Guam veterans, female veterans, and all Vietnam veterans. I became involved with the Vietnam Women's Memorial Foundation. In 1993 we placed the beautiful statue honoring women veterans of the Vietnam War. I have continued my involvement with the Vietnam Women's Memorial Foundation, and in 2023 we celebrate our 30th anniversary of the statue honoring all women who served during the Vietnam War.

As a Naval Reservist in 1990, I was recalled to active duty for Desert Shield/Desert Storm. At this time, I had my first anxiety attack! I could not imagine that I would have to go through this war trauma again, and now, with a young family to leave behind. Fortunately, I was sent to Washington, D.C., in an administrative role. My husband was called up to Bethesda Naval Hospital. Even though we didn't go overseas, we still had the anxiety of being on active duty during another war! It brought up all the old emotions of Vietnam! Today, I am a retired Navy nurse (for 35 years) and feel that I have successfully put that Vietnam part of my life in perspective. I love my Vietnam veterans, especially my Marines and my fellow Navy nurses. I am so proud and humble that I played a role in this very important part of American history. We did our jobs. We were not involved in politics about the war. We just did our jobs to the best of our ability, day in and day out. We came home with lots of scars and demons, but we dealt with them and carried on. Those who have never lived this experience have a difficult time understanding the impact of war. I have put this war experience to rest, but I know that there are so many that cannot move on, plus now we have more wars to process.

Patricia J. O'Hare

Patricia cared for American troops who had been POWs and severely injured while in captivity. Caring for American casualties laid the groundwork for a long naval career in trauma and emergency care.

I BECAME INTERESTED IN NURSING through the influence of my aunt. When I was a kid, I used to spend time looking through her old nursing school books. I was interested in medicine and nursing, so I followed in her footsteps. The school of nursing that she attended was later incorporated into Creighton University in Omaha, Nebraska. I attended the university from 1968 to 1972.

I ended up in the military purely by accident. A friend of mine in nursing was interested in joining the Army Nurse Corps upon graduation. She asked a recruiter to come talk to her in the dormitory. She wanted someone else to be in the room with her, so I agreed to be there. I became acutely interested when they mentioned paying for her tuition. In the end, she did not join the Army. I, however, looked into all three services. My plan was to eventually work on the goodwill ship *Hope* but two years of experience in nursing was required before working on the *Hope*. The Navy seemed a logical choice as a route to the *Hope*. I found the Navy uniforms much more attractive than the Army and Air Force. So, I signed on to the Navy Nurse Corps Candidate Program and had my last year of college paid for by the Navy.

My first choice for a duty station was Bethesda. I always heard about Bethesda being the hospital where the president of the United States went, so I thought it would be a good choice. I was granted my choice and loved everything about it.

I arrived at Bethesda in 1972. There was a shortage of nurses there, and a high percentage of my officer indoctrination class who had orders for Bethesda was placed directly into the intensive care unit. They were reluctant to put brand new graduate nurses into the ICU, but they had no choice. My ICU rotation in school was strong. That was actually where I wanted to be assigned, so I was happy with it. I learned more there than anywhere else in my career. I had excellent mentorship by nurses with extensive experience and willingness to share their knowledge. We also had a civilian nurse who was a pulmonary clinical nurse specialist and an excellent teacher. She was a wonderful person. She took the younger nurses under her wing and taught us everything she could.

There was an ICU residency program at Bethesda, so we were able to learn right along with the residents. A lot of the teaching took place at the bedside, and nurses were welcome to attend the classroom lectures for the residents. I spent many a day off in the classroom with the residents, soaking up all the knowledge I could absorb.

The patients in the ICU at Bethesda were critically ill. We provided all types of critical care: burn care, open heart surgery, severe head injuries, radical cancer surgeries, medical (non-surgical) critical illnesses, pediatric critical care, etc. Coronary care and transplant surgery were separate units from the ICU. Despite the acuity, I never burned out. I did eight years of critical care, 10 years of emergency department nursing and eventually moved into administration, but never grew tired of clinical bedside nursing. That's where my heart remains.

During the drawdown of the Vietnam War, I was at Bethesda when many POWs were released and brought home. I was working the ICU and recovery room (PACU) at the time. Many of the POWs required surgery for old fractures that had to be broken and realigned, so they came through the recovery room, post-surgery. Their injuries were severe. It made me angry that human beings were treated the way they were in captivity. They were kept in small cages and beaten severely. I still think about them, especially when I saw John McCain on TV, and think about what they endured. I don't know how they came out of that experience mentally sane and emotionally intact.

From Bethesda, I transferred to Philadelphia Naval Regional Medical Center in late 1975. There I gained more independence and autonomy, and used more of my own resources. I was the senior lieutenant and charge nurse in the ICU. It was a smaller hospital. There were few people to rely on. I remained there until 1977.

In 1977, the Navy was taking over the hospital in Okinawa, Japan, from the Army and I transferred there. I worked in the neonatal ICU (NICU) for 18 months. I had no experience in that area. But it was a great learning experience. With the exception of the ER doctor, there were generally no other physicians in-house at night. It was the ER physician who responded to any emergency we had in the NICU, or anywhere in the hospital, for that matter. In those days, there was no emergency medicine specialty. The ER was covered by all specialties, so it could be a dermatologist, radiologist, internist, surgeon or any specialist who would show up in an emergency. That was a bit scary, but we always got through it. We were the referral NICU for the Pacific, other than Tripler in Hawaii, so we cared for the most critical babies in our area of the Pacific. We had premature babies born at 24 weeks gestation; I would hold them in the palm of my hand. We grew very attached to them, and to their families, as they spent months in the NICU. My NICU experience was the first time I worked as the sole nurse, and had no one else to rely on. I learned to think ahead and anticipate, to be prepared for every situation, and to teach the corpsmen to do the same. Another new experience in Japan was working with the local nationals. We had Japanese nursing aides working in the newborn nursery who were outstanding, hardworking people. They were absolutely delightful. I still think of those ladies with fondness.

In Okinawa, I received orders back to Philadelphia. I was assigned to the emergency room. I tried telling the chief nurse that I was an ICU nurse, but she informed me that I was now an ER nurse. I ended up loving the ER more than I did critical care. It was a very busy ER. Every day the line of patients checking in was down the hall and out the door. The greatest skill I learned was triage. It was easy for a critically ill person to get lost in the long line of patients, so you had to be very aware of those waiting in line.

The Philadelphia ER was where I made the decision to specialize in emergency and trauma nursing and to make the Navy my career. Widener University in Chester, Pennsylvania, had a new master's degree program for clinical specialization in burns, emergency and trauma nursing. I began taking evening classes on my own time, then, applied and was selected for full time duty under instruction (DUINS). Upon graduation as a clinical nurse specialist, I was transferred to Little Creek Naval Amphibious Base, to the Admiral Joel T. Boone Clinic.

I was assigned to manage the ER at Boone Clinic, referred to as "Boone's Hospital," but it was just a branch outpatient clinic. Patients wanted ALL their care there, and would demand that ambulances take them to Boone Clinic regardless of their condition. We became adept at stabilizing critically ill patients and transferring them to the closest hospital. The ER there was probably worse than Philadelphia's ER. We often had only one nurse, sometimes two nurses during the day. There was only one night nurse and one physician. The ER was staffed by one nurse, one physician, one PA and several corpsmen. Again, the line of patients checking in usually extended down the hall to the door. We treated 100 to 130 patients daily—everything from minor illnesses and injuries to severe trauma, and even a victim of a small plane crash. There was never a moment's rest. But we enjoyed our work and provided superior care.

After four years at the Boone Clinic, I was transferred to the Naval Hospital Portsmouth where I worked as the clinical nurse specialist in the emergency department. When Desert Storm/Desert Shield began, I was moved to administration to fill in for the assistant director of nursing (she was deployed with Fleet Hospital 5), as well as the captain who did staffing for nursing service. I was an O-5 replacing two O-6s and I had wanted no part of administration. But flexibility is the name of the game. It was a very challenging time. We lost 700 hospital staff to the fleet hospital, and were backfilled with a lesser number of reservists—some of whom had not worked as nurses for a very long time. There were some steep learning curves on both sides of the fence. As a result of this reserve mobilization, things have changed considerably with reserve training and utilization. A much-needed change.

As I approached the 20-year mark, I put in my request and received my orders to retire. However, one evening as I walked out of the hospital I was overwhelmed by the feeling that I didn't want to retire. I realized that I didn't want to give up Navy nursing. I loved the Navy, loved the people, still loved the uniform and just couldn't walk away from it. So, the next morning, when the director of nursing arrived at 0530, I was there waiting for her. She asked, "Oh dear heart, what's the matter?" I said, "You're not going to believe this, but I don't want to retire." She and the commanding officer had tried their best to stop me from requesting retirement. Now I had to eat crow and ask for their assistance in getting the retirement orders rescinded. I was mortified, but the director of nursing just laughed and laughed and then went to bat for me. She spoke to the CO and the CO was successful in stopping my retirement orders. And, I was eternally grateful. I happily worked another six years as a nurse corps officer.

From Portsmouth, I was sent to Roosevelt Rhodes, Puerto Rico, as the director of nursing for two years. That was a 30–35 bed hospital with a large outpatient department supporting a huge base and several smaller distant bases. There was a large family housing area on base, so the hospital stayed very busy. I was blessed to have a staff of excellent nurses, especially those in leadership roles. Additionally, my executive officer was a nurse corps officer, so if I really needed leadership guidance, I could go to her.

From Puerto Rico, I returned to Naval Regional Medical Center, Portsmouth, Virginia, and worked for four years, until retirement. For those four years, I was department head of the critical care department and emergency department, as well as the corresponding outpatient clinics. It was a big job, but once again, I had outstanding nurses in leadership positions working for me, as well as stellar enlisted leadership. They made all my jobs easy.

After 18 months of retirement, I went back to work managing the trauma program at a local civilian hospital. One well recognized benefit of military nursing is that military nurses are taught to be leaders. Although my heart was at the bedside, I learned to be a manager and leader, as well. I was blessed to be able to spend most of my career where I wanted to be, in critical care and emergency nursing. But having the leadership and management experience, as well, gave me a leg up on the trauma program management position. The other unique aspect of military nursing is that you really have to become a teacher. There are constantly new corpsmen and nurses who have to be taught. In civilian nursing, turnover is slower. The requirement to be constantly teaching is not there. I learned a lot about improvisation and self-reliant leadership management. In the military, you don't have a choice but to be a leader. Now that I'm in civilian nursing, I can see the difference. Civilian nurses tend to find a niche and stay there. I was very fortunate, more than most military nurses. I spent most of my career where I loved it, in critical care and emergency nursing and at the bedside. By the time many become commanders, they were not in clinical roles anymore. I still was. You have to keep moving up the line because folks keep moving on. In civilian nursing, they stay there.

Faith played a part in my career. Raised a practicing devout Catholic, my faith was always there. I believe in a life after this world. Without that belief, I don't know how I would have coped with all the critical situations I dealt with, both in the military and now in civilian nursing.

Nancy J. Owen

I HAVE ALWAYS WANTED TO BE A NURSE. There were the traditional roles, nurses and teachers. I was Catholic so being a nun was a traditional role. I went to Catholic schools: grade school, high school, and nursing school. We were a middle-class family, so I didn't have a lot of money. Paying for nursing school was going to be a challenge. I graduated from high school in 1968. I worked for a year in a foam rubber factory, making the innards for wartime equipment, gluing straps on helmets and making inner bags for ambu bags. I worked at this same factory during my summers in high school. It was a little town, the town of York Haven, Pennsylvania. It had one of the old paper factories where everybody in the town worked.

I enrolled at St. Joseph's Hospital School of Nursing in Lancaster, Pennsylvania, thirty miles away from home. It was a long way in those days. I spent three years at St. Joe's nursing school, coming home many weekends. We lived in dormitories and had house mothers. I enjoyed it immensely and made so many good friends.

I think one of the poignant times during that first year was when the riots occurred at Kent State protesting the Vietnam War. Franklin-Marshall was a college about two blocks up the street. They had a peaceful march from their college to downtown Lancaster. We wanted to participate, but the school did not allow us to, so we all stood on our balconies and held candles and sang, *Let There Be Peace*. The seniors, being the rowdy ones, hung a peace sign on their dorms. The nuns were not too pleased about it. It wasn't that they didn't want us to think or have an opinion. It just wasn't appropriate, coming out of a religious institution, to even march in that peaceful march. The march really was peaceful. The whole thing about Kent State was very hard.

The Vietnam War was going on then, but I was very naïve about it. I had thought about going into the Navy. In fact, there was an article written up in our high school newspaper where they interviewed me about my future goals. Those goals were to become a nurse and join the

161

Navy. But, in my mind, I was going to be joining as a hospital corpsman and working my way through. Someone told me that it would be better if I got through nursing school, then joined and came in as an officer.

During my senior year, the recruiter came to the nursing school. The Navy was taking people with hospital diplomas at that time. She came to the school, by herself, and talked to people. There was another girl who was a good buddy of mine. After the talk and after we had gone home and thought about it, she said to me, "You know that doesn't sound like a bad idea. Would you want to go in, because they talked about the buddy system?" I thought it did sound like a good idea. I was from this little town in Pennsylvania and, other than going down to Rehoboth Beach, Ocean City, Atlantic City, I had never really been out of the state. I had never flown. Here it was 1972 and I was 21.

It was an overnight decision that both of us made. Four others from the school also decided to join the Navy. The nuns had no difficulty with that. I don't remember them having any opinion one way or the other. They allowed the recruiter to come in. There was nothing said to us at all. My dad always supported me in whatever I wanted to do. Mom was sick with breast cancer at the time. She was terminal, but I don't think I wanted to acknowledge that. Mom was also a paranoid schizophrenic. Things had been tough growing up in the house with that there.

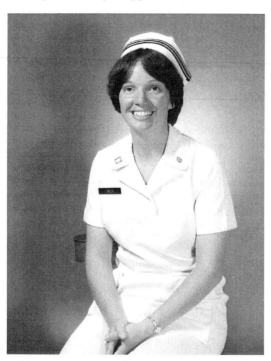

My friend and I went in on the buddy system. We went go off to Newport, Rhode Island, together and were guaranteed our first duty station together. We asked for Charleston, South Carolina, first on our list, and we got it. We wanted to go to Charleston because neither of us had ever been there before. It was at least on the same coast as Penn-

Lieutenant Nancy J. Owen during the Vietnam War conflict. Photo by permission.

sylvania. We wanted to go away, but wanted to be able to come home in some way. I remember packing up at home. I didn't pack a whole lot because I didn't have a whole lot.

I said goodbye to my mother. She died while I was at Newport. I came home when that happened. When I left home, I knew the end was near because she had metastasis. Dad was really strong. I had two brothers, one 10, the other 12, when she passed away. You know, when you try and take care of your own family members, it is tough. You become a family member, not a nurse. Even though I came home for a week, I was still able to finish with my own Newport class, even though we were only in Newport for five and a half weeks. That period of time is a little bit of a blur to me. I was away on liberty for the weekend when the call came that she had died. I was due back to stand the watch at the front desk. When I came back, people were kind of solemn and said, "Your roommate needs to see you." It was not my friend. They had put each of us in different rooms. It was my new roommate that told me. I remember somebody taking me to the Providence airport, which was an hour away, flying home, flying back.

This first trip up to Newport was a real experience. It was in September 1972. It was the first time I had ever flown and the plane was a real puddle jumper. We flew into the Providence, Rhode Island, airport. It is kind of a scary experience to fly for the first time, leave home and leave your family. My experience at Newport was very good. I became a company commander, even with that extra week away.

My friend and I finished our experience in Newport. We got to go home for a few days. Then we flew to Charleston. Neither of us had a car. The Air Force base and the airport shared a runway. We took a taxi to the BOQ. We kind of looked at ourselves on the steps of the BOQ and wondered, "What have we gotten ourselves into?" There we were with our suitcases and checking in at the front desk. At that time all the stewards were Filipino. They were very friendly and though sometimes they were difficult to understand, you got so you could understand them. So, here we were and they were kind of smiling at us. They said, "Oh, we will put you in the new wing."

They were very nice rooms. We had rooms across from each other. Later, we found out that we were two of 12 Navy nurses in the BOQ and there were probably 200 men, all types of groups from submariners to aviators to mostly shipboard. That has its pluses and minuses. We were from near Lancaster, smaller towns. While we had dated, it was not a lot. I left a boyfriend to go into the Navy. All of a sudden, I started getting asked out or having people knock on my door. You really didn't have much control because your door was not wide open, but available to anybody. So it was good and bad as far as the dating scene went. These guys were from places like Harvard and Yale. It was very flattering and kind of overwhelming to be asked out on so many dates. It had just never happened before.

We started out in the old Navy hospital in Charleston, South Carolina. It was a World War II vintage wooden hospital with the ramps. I referred to myself as a "ramp nurse." You covered four wards on the ramp. There was a sick officers' quarters, Charlie ward, echo, and foxtrot. Echo was the psych ward. Foxtrot was the medical ward. We had five major wards and some dependent wards.

St. Joe's was excellent preparation for the Navy. I learned an awful lot. I had a lot of skills and a lot of on-the-job kind of training. I felt pretty competent. However, the hospital corpsmen were very good at teaching us young nurses what was what. I owe them a lot. You really depended on them. We couldn't have done what we did without them.

We got people back from Vietnam and a lot of general surgical cases, like pilonidal cysts. That sticks in my mind because we just saw so many of those. There were no women on the ward, of course, just men. There were a couple of retirees. I remember one particular one because he was in a circo-electric bed. He was an older gentleman among all these young guys. This gentleman was probably in his '80s. Why I remember him most was because when we moved from the old hospital to the new hospital, he and I were the last ones to go. They took all the other people first. So, when we got ready to go, I said, "Joe, it is just you and me." I packed up the medicine boxes and Joe and away we went. This was in early 1973. I hadn't been there very long. I arrived in November 1972.

I do remember President Nixon announcing the pullout of troops from Vietnam. I remember all the guys with their overbed tables with little black and white TVs. I remember that the whole ward went silent, just silent. You could have heard the proverbial pin drop. You could see all these guys, who had been in Vietnam at one time or another, just looking at these TVs. Some were in tears, some with looks of disbelief. Others were, I think, angry. Not a word was spoken. There were a lot of mixed emotions. I felt very neutral. I was still very naïve. It was a very controversial time to come into the Navy. I had learned a trade and wanted the skills I had learned to take care of people. That was my reason to come into the Navy. It didn't matter to me if there was a war or not. I knew I wouldn't have to go to Vietnam, now that the troops were being pulled out. I knew that Navy nurses had to have one tour of duty under their belt before being able to go Vietnam. This was unlike our

Army cohorts, who went straight over. But that didn't even weigh in on my decision to go into the Navy, I wanted to serve my country. There was this patriotic part of me that wanted to serve. When the pullout was announced I just remember the silence.

I wasn't part of the hippie or drug scene before I went into the service. I considered myself very conservative. I had lived in a small town and had been going to the Catholic schools. I did have a boyfriend when I was young. I was 14. There was an older fellow. I worked in a little soda fountain not even a block away from the house. I met him there. He was a little older, about 20, and was very nice. The reason I bring him up is he was sent to Vietnam. He joined the Army, went to Fort Benning for jump school. I was probably about 16 when he was injured very badly. We were still going together. I had a ring and everything. He had gone off to war. I remember his parents taking me to Valley Forge Army Hospital, near Philadelphia, to see him. When he left, he had been 5'10", 180 lbs. When I saw him at Valley Forge, he was probably 110 lbs. He had shrapnel in his spine. He was alert and oriented. He wasn't on any kind of life support or anything. But it was also at a time when my concern for him as a boyfriend was waning. I had found other people. I felt very bad because I returned his ring that day. I think back on that. Afterwards, my going in the Navy was kind of to make up for that. I didn't think in those terms, but I felt bad about doing that. His being injured put a face on the war, a returning person from the war, somebody I knew. He knew I had gone in the military because he was still around town. Some pictures and an article about me surfaced in the local paper. I'm sure that he was probably aware. He survived to come back to our hometown. I tried to talk to him, but he was changed and didn't want to talk about the war too much.

Another important thing that happened in Charleston was that I met my husband. Many nurses were dating men from Charleston. He was a supply officer on a submarine. He would fly over to Scotland with the Gold crew. He would be out for six months and in for six months. When he was in, he was home based in Charleston. When he was out, he was with the submarine. The laundry room was by his room. One time, I was coming back from the laundry room. I must have met him before because he invited me in for a piece of chocolate cake. We struck up a conversation. Another thing was that you dressed up a little more when you ate your meals in the BOQ. It was neat because you met a whole different group of people each meal. If you wanted to go in with your friends, you just kind of walked in together and they would seat you together. It was a real community. We really dressed up pretty nicely, not just because the men were there, but because that was the thing you did. You might remember the palazzo pants, the sort of flowing mid-leg pants with blouses and sweaters over the top. I remember going out when we got a little money in our pockets. It was a nice thing to do.

We started dating and became engaged in 1973. We married in October 1974 in Charleston, South Carolina, at the little Eternal Father of the Sea Chapel there. Three of my four bridesmaids married men that they had met at the BOQ. It was quite a place. Sometimes I wonder where I would be if I hadn't lived there. It was just in the blueprint. We were both active duty and were pretty much able to have our duty stations together. We looked ahead to see what was available for supply and nursing and didn't ask for the impossible. We did take separations throughout our career, but in general, we did pretty well for being a dual military couple. Interestingly enough, he was scheduled to go to Scotland the month after we were married and do a turnaround with a new supply officer that was coming on board. We were going to live in the BOQ, even though we were married. They gave us a two-room suite there because they knew we were going to leave in January to go to Portsmouth, Virginia, together. Normally your duty stations were for three years. They were going to give me no cost orders because I hadn't done the three years, and there wasn't an opening in Portsmouth. However, any possessions we had went with my husband's orders, so, no cost orders were not a big deal.

I bought my first car in Charleston. It was a butterscotch pinto. I paid $2,000 brand new. There was a warrant officer that lived next to me in the BOQ. You always want to take someone else with you when you are going out to buy a car. So, he helped me with my car. I kept mine for ten years.

I was in Charleston from 1972 until January 1975. Then, we moved to Portsmouth, Virginia. I was stationed at the old naval hospital, which was 14 or 15 stories high. My husband worked over at Norfolk at the air station there. I worked on W14, the women's surgical ward. It was a fabulous experience. I worked there the whole time I was in Portsmouth, from 1974 to 1977. We had a unique group of nurses, hospital corpsmen and civilians. We really gelled and worked so well together to take care of those patients.

I remember one of the nurses we called Admiral Toots. She would go around and be whipping these women into shape. She would say, "Now honey, you know you got to do this and you got to do that." She had also been a nun. I have known a couple of nurses during my career who had been nuns and who had come into the Navy. We had really good times. She was the kind of person you would have coffee with at two in the morning. You could talk to her about anything and every-thing. She was older coming into the Navy because she had been in the convent. I think she was a lieutenant.

I made lieutenant at Portsmouth. During Vietnam, people made rank fairly quickly. It seemed that every time I was up for the next rank, they would push the date back. At one time, they were going from ensign to JG in twelve months, but then it went from fifteen to eighteen months. It took me the longer time to make JG and two years to make lieutenant.

By 1975, we weren't seeing any war injuries. The wards were not open wards. They had individual rooms, two to a room. On the 14th floor, when the ships would come down the river, you could see the ships' superstructures at about eye level. It was a hardworking group. We were still doing the old routine: seven nights, three or four days off and seven PMs, same as in Charleston. Though, in Portsmouth, it seemed like those nights rolled around about once a month. In Charleston, you didn't feel like you could ask for a particular day off. When Wayne would come back from deployment, he would come back on a Friday night. If I was due to work that night, I wouldn't even consider asking for the time off. You could switch with someone, but things were pretty strict—e.g., the straight-across haircuts and the starched white uniforms. The pant suits came out while I was at Portsmouth. That was a real revolution, the pant suit with the cap. I really probably gained a lot of knowledge and confidence in myself at Portsmouth. I became charge nurse there. You became charge nurses very quickly and at a young age. You didn't need commanders on the wards to be senior nurses.

I was in Portsmouth from 1975 to 1977 when both my husband and I got orders to the Philippines. That was a short time at the Portsmouth duty station, but I think they probably needed people overseas. The Philippines was probably one of the best tours ever, just the whole cultural aspect of it. We called the Philippines' Cubi Point "Jungle General." It was up on a hill and through the jungle. Subic Bay was down along the water front. They were within just a few miles of each other. People would ask if you were stationed at Subic or Cubi. Cubi was the hospital, but it was called Naval Hospital Subic Bay.

We were married, so we got quarters on the base at Sangley Loop. These were houses that had been floated down from the old Sangley Loop near Manila. We had maids and house boys. They were beautiful houses in pristine condition and well maintained. The senior nurse and single nurses still lived in nurses' quarters right next to the hospital. It was almost like going back to the dormitories at St. Joe's. Because so many married nurses were coming, they closed that hospital quarters, made it corpsmen's barracks and moved the single nurses into the BOQ, which was actually at Cubi.

Talk about an experience in baptism by fire. Seventeen nurses are all we had over there. We had 80 to 100 beds. It almost reminded me a little of the ramps because you had a surgical, psych, and medicine ward and an emergency room. You were the only nurse on duty, and you carried five sets of keys. There was one hospital corpsman on each of those wards. You never knew what was coming up the hill. You would get a call that somebody was coming in from town. It was rough out in town. People would drink. They were young guys and would get themselves in all kinds of trouble. On paydays they would be found unconscious and be brought to the hospital. One of the ones I remember wasn't outside the base. He was actually on base. His motorcycle caught the end of a post that was going across the bridge and caught him right in his skull. He was basically dead when he got to the emergency room. To get someone, even from the housing area, which is where he was, up to the emergency room, was a good twenty minutes. We lost the golden time there.

Unusual things would happen. The locals would cut the phone lines from downtown up to the hospital. The money they would get for the copper they could take out of the phone lines would support the family for a year. Our phone communication would be cut. There was an ambush in town between the New People's Army, kind of a left-wing rebel group, and some of the locals. Normally, we wouldn't be taking care of Philippine nationals. In this case, there were several injuries, so we had people from both factions on the same ward. They called in the Marines, for just this incident, to protect the hospital. They were afraid that someone from either side was going to come in and kill someone from the other side. Normally, we didn't have much security at all.

Superstitions were very strong in the Philippines. There was one about a white lady being close to the hospital. If you ever mentioned to a cab driver anything about a white lady, he would drop you off and leave. Supposedly, a nurse had been killed many years ago and her spirit is still there. We even had an exorcism performed one time. All the civilian nurses refused to come to work because they thought the GYN spaces were haunted. The chaplain actually came up and performed an exorcism. He had to do it to get the nurses to come back to work. I was at the hospital during the time, but I did not actually witness the exorcism.

We had these big bull monkeys that would chase people. Some people would go jogging but the bull monkeys would chase them. You had to run fast and carry a big stick. If you showed dominance to them, they would somewhat back off, but they were huge. You would see them when you drove to work. We had big boars and big fruit bats. I was working the medicine wards one day, early in the morning. The sky was kind of dark and I could see these bats flying outside the window. I felt like I was in the Wizard of Oz. There were just tons of them. It was the first time I had seen them. It truly was a jungle.

You saw medical conditions that you had only read about. We had one case of coccidioidomycosis. You saw malaria and cholera and we treated those conditions. You talk about the classic rice water stools. People died from cholera because they would get so dehydrated. Also, that was before we had all the equipment for cardiac monitoring. It was probably my first introduction to cardiac nursing. A good friend and someone I consider a mentor was there. She taught me all I needed to know to take care of people with chest pain. I went to a couple of classes at Clark Air Force Base, which was about an hour away. They presented educational classes. I took a cardiac care class. Eventually in my career, I became charge nurse at Balboa, San Diego Naval Medical Center, on the coronary care unit. It was kind of a preparation.

But on this medicine ward, in addition to the cardiac patients, we had people with hepatitis. Some of the hepatitis patients turned so yellow they were almost green. A lot of the hepatitis was due to tattoos. They go off ships in Hong Kong and get tattooed. I'd ask them if they went to Ricky's or Pinky's. Their eyes would get big as saucers. We had heard that these were the two establishments that weren't using the cleanest of needles. They'd ask, "How did you know that?" We saw an awful lot of venereal disease. Gonorrhea (GC) was rampant in the Philippines. I remember a fellow with GC tonsillitis. Here they were eighteen or nineteen years old and in the hospital being treated with IV antibiotics. I would give them my five-dollar lecture. "Now, honey, do you know how you got this?" "No, ma'am." So, we would proceed to talk about that. They were so naïve. It was their first time in the Navy. It was probably their first time to be out on the town. I do remember that in the Philippines, the men started building up resistance to the medications for GC. One of the things they did to counteract the social problems, because we knew the guys were going to go out, no questions asked, was that we had social clinics. You actually had card carrying prostitutes. They would get examined, get treated and be given a card to carry. So, I guess you could ask if your prostitute had been seen before you had any kind of sexual relations. That probably didn't happen, but at least we had a little bit of control that way, a little bit of impact on the community.

I saw my first and only case of leprosy while I was over there. I remember the doctor showing us this lesion. It almost looked like a vaccination mark. The skin was kind of pulled a little bit. He didn't have a lot of other symptoms. But the doctor being astute, was able to recognize that. Of course, we now have treatment for leprosy. This patient was a military person and had family in the Philippines there. I remember him being treated. I'm not sure how widespread leprosy was in the Philippines. I know that TB was endemic. Certainly, anyone coming back from there would have to be treated.

I'm sure there are many more stories I could tell. Over there you worked hard together and you played together. If you needed to see a doc, you found yourself being examined by the doc you worked with. It was just that close knit because there are so few of us. We had two general surgeons, a couple of medicine doctors, one or two psych, one GYN. I don't remember any Filipino doctors. Certainly, there were Filipino nurses. They worked mostly on the civilian wards. We did have a pediatrician. You pulled OR as your duty. You didn't have the NOD, nurse of the duty, but you would get called for OR duty a couple of times a month. Inevitably you would get called for a cesarean section. You would circulate. Your corpsmen, your OR techs were wonderful. I remember a helicopter going down in Mindanao, one of the southern provinces, full of Marines. Fifteen of them went to Clark Air Base. We had three of them come to us and all three of them needed to be in the operating room. So, you got called in. It was baptism by fire there. You really became a general practitioner. Charting was minimal at that time. The corpsmen did a lot of the charting.

The other patient I remember from over there was one with acromegaly. I was coming onto night duty and it was all dark with that little bit of light at the nurses' station. I was kind of warned about this gentleman, that some of his features were a little grotesque. I am sitting there, reading something and he came up to the nurses' station. I just remember this huge head with these bushy eyebrows that were pulled kind of taut, the large forehead feature and the huge hands. He was really a gentle giant.

I remember the Seal team guys. We had a great Seal team over there. The guys were just a whole different breed. They would just protect you to the nth degree. Well, one of them was working with underwater explosives. It went off very close to his femoral artery. It didn't hit the femoral artery, but he was recuperating on the surgical floor. He had a pretty good hole in his leg. He was quite a practical jokester. The doctors and nurses would go up and say, "I need to take a look at your wound." He had this ketchup bottle with a string on it that he would squirt you with. He was a practical jokester, but the most wonderful person. He was there over Christmas time. He would help me wheel people to the operating room. He had his little khaki shorts on, the Seal team shorts, the ever-present blue and white striped hospital gown and a ball cap.

One night his other Seal team buddies came in and stole him off the ward to take him for a six pack. You kind of allowed more than you ever would in this day. We have been very good friends ever since. He retired as a master chief. Later on, when I went to Croatia, he came to the airport to see me off and gave me something to put in my pocket as a good luck charm. He is a very good wood carver. It was a beautiful piece of iron wood about two inches by four inches, just a block of wood beautifully polished and carved. The relationships you make just last forever.

My husband left the Philippines first because he was going to Monterey to postgraduate school. This was one of those separations. There wasn't anything for me up there. I wanted to go back to get my bachelor's degree. I took several general education classes while I was in the Philippines. My school of nursing did not affiliate with any college, so I really had no college credits. I was kind of starting from ground zero, but really wanted to get that bachelor's degree. I took several classes and then applied for duty under instruction (DUINS), and was accepted. I applied for a couple of schools: San Jose, thinking that would be reasonably close to Monterey, but not really. Then, University of San Diego (USD) and was accepted. I think the Navy chose University of San Diego, which in the end, turned out to be very good. I knew that I could come to the hospital there after that. There were plenty of duty stations for my husband to come to after he finished his duty in Monterey in 15 months. After he left, they made me move out of our house in the Philippines and stay in the BOQ because I was, then, unaccompanied.

I came back to San Diego, got an apartment by myself because my husband was up in Monterey. It took me three years to get my bachelor's because I didn't have any previous classes. The Navy paid for those three years. At that time, you could take that long. I don't think they will pay for more than two years now. I think at University of San Diego they have the bachelor's to master's program. In that case they can stay longer.

I went over to the amphibious base to do my clinical. My first patient was a dolphin. I wondered how I would tell my civilian instructors that my first patient was a dolphin. Of course, the Seal team uses those animals for mine retrieval. My exam read, "Skin—gray, wet to touch." Only in the military could you get these kinds of experiences. They brought him in to do an x-ray because he wasn't eating. I remember them swabbing the floor and kind of putting a harness on the dolphin to get it out of there. Only in the Navy.

I finished DUINS. My husband came to San Diego to work in the supply center after 15 months in Monterey. I graduated from USD summa cum laude and went to work at Balboa, the pink palace. I have a shirt with that on it. This was 1982. I was assigned to the coronary care unit and was going to be taking over that unit. I really didn't think I had the skills, so I went through several classes. The unit was very comfortable with the previous charge nurse who had been there. They were not really comfortable with me coming in and not having the experience. So, I really felt that I needed to hone those skills and prove myself in doing the job. I learned my job very well. Clinical-wise, I think that was the highlight of my career to work there in that unit and take care of those patients. They were really near and dear to my heart. The emergency room was down on the ground floor. So, they would bring them up. They had to take them outside and you would hear them kind of going, "clank, clank, clank" to come down over the sidewalk to 9–1 North. The CCU was moved to Building 26. We stayed there until the move into the new hospital in 1988. I left in 1986, before they made the move into the new hospital.

In 1984, I became pregnant. It was a wonderful pregnancy. At that time there weren't a whole lot of women pregnant in the Navy. I came in the Navy in 1972 when you could be married, but not pregnant. In 1973 was the first time that if you became pregnant you were allowed to stay in. So, by 1984 a lot of people were pregnant, but still a lot of provisions were not there. I worked until the day I delivered. I felt good. I was charge nurse in the coronary care unit.

I remember standing inspection. There were no rules that you didn't have to stand inspection. "Dress that line. Oh, you can't dress that line." I was standing personnel inspection a week before I delivered. I was at home when I started into labor. Here I am calling into the labor deck and asking them if they're busy. "Well, we were earlier, but not so much now."

I had a normal vaginal delivery. It was a wonderful experience, having all the people around that you know. I was in labor about 14 hours. My husband deployed to Acapulco, and made it back about 24 hours before the delivery. I had to go back to work in four weeks. If you had a C-section you got to be off six weeks. I breast-fed as much as I could, for six to eight weeks. I felt like my son had a good start. In terms of childcare, I had a very wonderful woman from church. I was very active in church over in Coronado, the Sacred Heart Church. This woman had been a friend before. She had taken in other children, but Paul was the only child she was going to be taking in at this time. What a wonderful gift. That just lifted such a weight off my shoulders. She was tremendous.

I had in-laws that lived there as well. That enabled us to live through our jobs, continue our careers and have a family. It all worked out.

In 1986, I left San Diego and went to Philadelphia Naval Hospital. During Vietnam, it was the amputee center and a very busy place. But, in 1986, things were really kind of gearing down. There was a question about whether it was going to be on the BRAC list. They were even headed toward closure. The shipyard and other activities around Philadelphia were kind of phasing out. My husband got stationed at Willow Grove Naval Air Station. I got stationed at the hospital. We kind of took a map, put a pin between and ended up living in Langhorne, Pennsylvania. It was 45 minutes to an hour drive for both of us. The shipyard had childcare. I would take Paul in the mornings and drop him off at the childcare. Five minutes away was work.

I worked in the emergency room at Philadelphia. We didn't take trauma in that emergency room. There were plenty of other places in Philadelphia that did trauma, like Jefferson and Temple. Although we had 12 floors there, very few wards were open. It really started tapering off until we had less than 20 inpatients. Our focus really became outpatient ambulatory care. Also, in kind of this phasing out of the hospital, we got word that we were going to close the emergency room. We were literally out there taking the sign down when we got an order to leave the sign up. We got these t-shirts that said, "I survived the closing of Philadelphia Naval Hospital, and the opening, and the closing, and the opening...." It was really kind of awkward and unsettling. As we downsized, they did keep the emergency room open. I became the department head of ambulatory care: the emergency room and the ambulatory care clinics.

As we downsized, we would take on extra jobs. I became double-hatted, as the public affairs officer. At a time when there was a lot of public affairs to do, I had no training. Fortunately, there was a real public affairs officer over at the shipyard to help me. So, speaking of strange things, between the dolphin being my first patient and the first day of me being the public affairs officer, I got a call wanting to know if I knew anything about the missing feet found about a block away from the hospital. They appeared to be human feet. I thought somebody was pulling my leg, no pun intended. Come to find out, they were primate feet and were perhaps from a veterinary school in Philadelphia. My response was, "We dispose of our body parts properly. No, these are not ours." The second issue I had to deal with was my own oil spill. This was probably a year and a half after the Valdez oil spill in Alaska. There was some type of oil spill across from the hospital. I had to deal with that.

On the positive side of things, I had a friend who headed the orthotic shop that had been there as part of the Vietnam era. He had polio as a child. He had learned the trade of making orthotics because when he would go in to be refitted for a brace, the person making the brace would tell him that it was going to take "X" amount of time. My friend would say, "Well, what if I helped you? Could I get my brace sooner?" That is how he learned his trade. He did the most wonderful job. He would fabricate the most wonderful orthotics and booties, particularly for the orthopedic patients. I did a whole article on him for the local newspaper. I took the pictures and wrote the article. It appeared in one of the local newspapers back there. He was just tremendous. He was one of the last orthotic folks. Philadelphia was kind of out there ahead, as far as prosthetics were concerned. Philadelphia and Oakland were the two Navy orthotic centers, but Oakland closed. Philly was the only one left.

Philadelphia ended up on the base closure list. We were surprised because we were already in the process of downsizing. I received many phone calls that day, people wanting to have our equipment. It is so funny how people react to that list. It is just a list when it first comes out. There haven't been any decisions made. I get all these media calls and they wanted to meet with me or a representative from the hospital. The word from Washington was to make no comment. I had 25 reporters who wanted some information. I called our public affairs officer at the shipyard. Between the two of us we decided that we would have a press conference at 11:00 in the morning. This was my first press conference. We had it in the CO's conference room. I had a prepared statement. I planned to get up and read my prepared statement. I walked into the CO's conference room. There were probably 25 people and ten microphones sitting up front. They started firing questions. You don't get your statement out. All they heard was that we had 13 patients in this 12-story building. It seemed like quite a waste. Yet, in the ambulatory care area we still had a lot of patients and we were still doing a service. Of course, we had an antiquated building. Anyway, I had an ally on the *Philadelphia Inquirer* and he kind of said, "Why don't you let her answer one question at a time." You learn who your allies are. He kind of stayed later and found out what was really going on. So, that was sort of my debut. You ask yourself, "What am I going to be doing in the Navy?" It is always more than you expected when you came out of nursing school.

After Philadelphia, I went back to school again. In 1989, I went back to the University of Pennsylvania to get a master's in critical care. The positive note about the clinical master's was that it was only a year and had no thesis attached, kind of unusual. I loved it because there was a very small group of us, 15 in our particular program. However, the administrative master's would have also kept me in sync with my husband's tour. I finished up my clinical master's. When I was ready for reassignment, he had another year to finish in Philadelphia.

I got orders back to San Diego. We had bought a condo in Coronado and had always rented it out. My son and I moved back and lived in it. My in-laws helped out with childcare. We were very fortunate in 1976 when we were on our way to the Philippines. We bought into the high-rise condos in Coronado. That was our foot in the door. It was a stretch to pay $100,000 for something, but in 1976 that was what it was.

I worked in San Diego in the new hospital in 1990. I worked on the med-surg floor as a clinical nurse specialist. There wasn't anything in critical care at the time. Eventually, I worked as the assistant department head in critical care: SICU, CCU, and the transition unit. I did that for a couple of years. Then they tapped me to be the patient relations person: special assistant to the admiral for patient relations, commonly called the complaint department. We handled the Congressional inquiries. I was also a liaison to the United Veterans Council, a group of veterans' organizations. I continue to be involved with them at the former chapel to the Navy hospital. It is now a veterans' museum and memorial in Balboa Park in San Diego, which is fantastic.

I was working in that position when the XO came in my office in November 1993. He closed the door and said, "We've got a mission." He said, "We are going to Croatia." I think I did realize that there was a war going on in Bosnia, but we didn't realize that there had been another field hospital over there. As bits and pieces came through, they told us that we were going to be going in with the Air Force, who had been there. The Army had been there before and set up a MASH unit in Zagreb on the tarmac at the airport.

We were to go in March, so the wheels started churning. We weren't allowed to say anything to our family at first. A month later we were given permission to tell our families because you had to prepare. We trained together in the coldest January at Camp Pendleton. We froze in those wooden structures and tents. We had trained before as kind of a partial unit, but when we got the orders to go, we really trained. We had to bring in some extra people to fill some extra billets. Ten years before this, if you had said to me, "You're in the Navy. You are going to be going to Croatia," I would have said, "I don't think so."

I knew where Croatia was. Both my grandparents came over from Croatia in the early 1900s. My maiden name was Knezic. My father was born there. I don't think the XO knew that. He knew what my background was from a clinical and military standpoint. He chose me to be the director of nursing. He was going as the commanding officer. We had a terrific group of people that were from the command.

In March 1994, Fleet Hospital 6 boarded a plane out of North Island. We were going over in three waves. We were the first wave. We had a person on the ground there telling us what we needed, what kind of personnel we needed. We were kind of doing this by the seat of our pants. Although we trained for the actual fleet hospital, we weren't going to have to set one up. It was already there. I started communicating with the senior Air Force nurse there. We started getting some situational reports from our man on the ground. He was medical service corps and kind of a bean counter. We found when we got there that we could have used a little bit different mix of personnel. Everybody that went to Croatia volunteered to go. We had 21 nurses that we took over. We had a total of 130 people. In addition to that, we had Seabees that went over and helped us with construction and maintenance. We also had a contingent of Marines from Camp Lejeune who provided our security.

In addition to our fleet hospital training, we did train on weapons. We went up to Camp Pendleton, on a rainy afternoon, with our 9mm weapons because there was a chance we would have to use them. We had an armory. We could check out those weapons if we were going on a mission away from Zagreb or if we needed to defend our camp. Normally, medical personnel are non-combatant. We don't use weapons. The people who are going to the Gulf now are being issued weapons, which is a whole change in thinking. I had been through the C4 and C4A schools in San Antonio with some background in trauma and ACLS. It had been quite a while since I had actually done some clinical things. I was going over as the director of nursing.

It was a very long flight. Washington, D.C., Dover and then straight over to Zagreb. We just stopped to fuel. When we arrived in Zagreb, we were met by the Air Force and members of the joint task force who were there. Several of our members slept in a large tent called RUBB Hall the first night. Much to my dismay, the former chief nurse had already departed, no turnover. I did get to sleep in what was to become my personal hootch. We had several orientation classes and a tour of the camp. Camp Pleso was the name of the camp. I think we had prepared ourselves to see gunshot wounds. As it turned out, there were very few such wounds. We saw land mine injuries. I don't believe we had prepared ourselves physically or mentally for that scenario. We knew they were there, but until we got there and started seeing some of those, we didn't realize how devastating they could be. If they were alive, they most likely had lost a limb or something. Seeing the injuries for the first time really affected us.

We had some classes about land mines. The French were the land mine experts. They were the ones who had to go out and make sure areas were free of land mines. They would do this with bayonets. They couldn't do it with metal detectors because there was no metal in the land mines. They would put flak vests on and helmets and go out with bayonets and stick them into the ground. Our ambulance would stand by on duty with them. We had a couple of casualties from people who were actually trying to detect the mines. The whole area was mined from the previous 1991

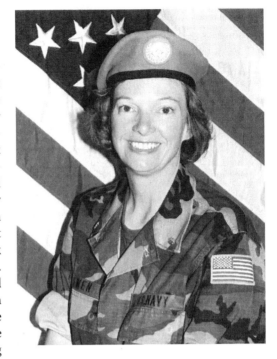

Commander Nancy J. Owen in NATO uniform in Bosnia. Photo by permission.

conflict between Yugoslavia and Croatia. Even around our camp were areas that had mine signs on them, "Stay on the sidewalks." You know how you do certain things when you come back from a war? I stayed on the sidewalks for a while, even after I came back. It got just kind of stuck in your head.

The rest of the place was pretty civilized. We had liberty and could go out in town on the buddy system. We were able to go out to restaurants and things. We were there under the UN and all wore the blue beret, which some people felt was controversial. We wore the UN patch on one arm and the American flag on the other. This was the United Nations peacekeeping force, Operation Provide Promise. To our knowledge, it was the first UN mission that Navy nurses were really on. We were there with 26 other nations: French, Pakistanis, Norwegians, Finnish, Canadians, Swedes, Dutch, Russians and several others. Each contingent had their own camp. The U.S. had the greatest number of women, about 25. Our main mission was to care for the United Nations troops. We were not there to care for the Bosnians or Croatians. We were there to support 40,000 United Nations troops throughout Croatia and

Bosnia. We were not the only medical group,but one of the largest there at Zagreb. The other contingents had smaller medical groups, some stationed in other areas of Yugoslavia: Tuzla, Sarajevo. Even though we were supposed to be a MASH unit, we would end up being a tertiary hospital. We kept people much longer in Zagreb than we did in Vietnam when people were medevacked out very quickly.

One of our first patients was a Russian hurt in a mine accident. If he had gone back to Russia, he might not have gotten the care because of facilities. We followed him to the point where he was fitted with a prosthesis. He wanted to go back to his unit. He ended up going back as a unit clerk. He was in our camp for almost our whole tour. One of the neatest things to see was him riding his bicycle with his prosthetic leg toward the end of our time there. We were there for six months from March 1994 to August 1994. We were replaced by another Navy group, Fleet Hospital 5 out of Norfolk, Virginia. The Army had been there for two tours, Air Force one and then it was the Navy's turn.

We had people with interesting diseases. We had UN people with mumps and measles. People from lots of different groups coming because they thought the UN would give them uniforms. Some countries accepted stipends to come, actually got paid a salary. We were not allowed to do that. That would have made us mercenaries. We got paid our regular salary plus a little extra for combat pay. The others were considered mercenary just by the definition of a mercenary being a soldier paid by another country. The Pakistanis were the most unusual. By day they wore combat uniforms, but by night they were in their traditional garb. They had their traditional camps. They were not used to seeing women. Here we were in our camouflage, covered, and in some cases, in civilian clothes. We would be walking by and their eyes were all on us. Some people were very uncomfortable with that. So, they asked me what we could do. I said, "Well, I will call the State Department and talk with them." We had all these communications capabilities. I did call and was told to just ignore them. However, one day one of the nurses was walking by. They were staring. She just looked at them and said, "boo." I don't think they were expecting that. It didn't change anything. They still would stare. Now, we were in the Middle East, having to cover up and observe their cultural mores.

Each contingent had a different assignment. The French were the mine people. The people from the Netherlands would transport people. They transported a lot of the goods down to Bosnia. They had big convoys of trucks. The Norwegians were in charge of dispatching the airplanes and loading and unloading people and cargo from the planes. There was this sea of planes and vehicles all painted white with UN on them. The first thing you saw on the tarmac was this lineup. All containers around our hospital were white with UN on them. There were all these different makes and models of planes we had never seen before, some Russian planes. How could you prepare? You just didn't know what to expect. Half of the hospital was under a hangar. The other half, including the emergency room and all of our tent city living area, was out in the open. Fortunately, we were there from March to August, unlike our predecessors who had been there during the snow. The climate and latitude were about the same as Pennsylvania. The summer would get fairly warm. In the winters, they would get snow. They weren't prepared for pulling snow off the tents.

As for the tents, I had a little hooch that was probably eight by ten feet inside a large tent that could sleep 10–12 people. We all kind of personalized our space in whatever way we could: things from home, things from the Air Force. You always want to follow the Air Force. The fleet hospital usually has cots. We had regular beds because the Air Force personnel had been able to get lots of things sent to them, including regular twin beds with mattresses. I had my "wardrobe," obtained from the nurse whom I relieved. It was one of those plastic things that you use to carry your clothing in. It had a place to put all your little things and some pockets on it. It made a little closet. I had a coffee pot. We had a little PX. There was a general PX that carried everything from Mozart Chocolates to liquor. We had our officers' club. The Norwegians had what they called a Bunker Bar, an old bunker made into a general meeting place where they celebrated their national holidays.

I spoke before about my roots in Croatia. My paternal grandparents came over from Croatia in the early 1900s to Ellis Island. I knew that my grandmother sent money to a granddaughter in Croatia, so I knew that there was still family. I knew her name and her address. We had a physician from Croatia in the emergency room that helped us with translation and interacted between us and the civilian community. He was able to locate my family. As it turned out, we ended up going to visit my cousin. She lived about 30 miles away from the camp. We had to take some security because where she lived was right on the border of Croatia and Bosnia. The security people gladly went on this excursion with us. It was kind of a publicity thing because we took press and public affairs people along. We spent some time with my cousin and her family in their Croatian home. I still keep in touch with her through letters and email.

We were able to go out into the hospitals in Zagreb. We visited with the nurses there and saw what they had or didn't have. Zagreb was better off than Sarajevo and some of the other towns. They still had a pretty good infrastructure in Zagreb. It is just that their supplies were running so short. We were there in a peacekeeping mode and to provide some care. They took care of their own military and civilians who got injured.

We were what was called a third echelon hospital. We were to get people taken care of and medevacked to wherever they came from. We ended up taking care of some of these people all the way to rehab stage, such as the Russian soldier mentioned previously. It was only through association with the hospitals in Zagreb that we were able to do this. The beds that we had were not beds that you could raise the heads. They were regular cots, pretty much. We had to get our Seabees to make some things that would help us get the heads up. We would tell them what we wanted. True to their motto "CAN DO," they always came through with what was needed. They were incredible in what they could make and take care of for us. It is amazing how we can adapt. Each deployment is different but, in many ways, they are similar experiences. They are unique in what you have to adapt and conquer to provide the care.

You don't go over to a war zone thinking you have to put people in isolation. We had people from other countries who did not receive normal childhood immunizations. We had people with mumps and measles. Yet we had a field situation in a field hospital where you had no positive pressure. We tried our best to isolate a couple of the people we had, but it didn't work very well. Again, we were getting the Seabees to try to help us out with some fans blowing against this door. It would, at least, keep the air in and not circulating in the rest of the hospital The whole time we were there, the creativity was amazing.

Dental care for many of the people from third world countries was nonexistent. A couple of dental officers would bring somebody in to take care of a tooth that was hurting. They would find a whole mouthful of decay and other problems. I think it was a priority issue. Someone from Britain, Norway or Sweden had more access. We pulled a record number of teeth. What was interesting for our group was that normally, in any kind of war, the number of admissions is more related to disease or medical problem than injury. When the Air Force or Army was there, they had about a 30 to 60 percent disease-related admissions to injury-related. We had 52 percent injury-related admissions to 48 percent disease admissions. The only thing we could figure out was that every three months the new troops from other countries were brought into the theater. These were consignment soldiers. They were signed up for X amount of time. These were not career military. Each of them had to do their stint in the military. Not being familiar with the land mines and terrain, there would be more injuries from the land mines or from motor vehicle accidents. We probably had more inpatients than previous groups. That was probably because we sought to go after and open up more care. Troop numbers increased to 40,000 troops from what may have been 20,000 or 30,000 earlier on. They were from 26 different nations. It was unbelievable.

The other challenge was that they didn't all speak a common language. We were field testing some new equipment or new technology. We had a "universal translator." The problem was that you could ask the question in the person's own language, but when the person would answer back it couldn't interpret the answer. So, you could ask yes or no questions, but you were limited to that. Many of the other nations would be able to speak a couple of different languages. You would have somebody who spoke Norwegian and German and someone who would speak German and English. The Norwegians could almost all speak some English. The Finnish troops had a unique language that was difficult for most of the other countries, but there were a few who spoke English. Even the Norwegians didn't understand the Finns.

A lot of these contingents had some basic medical care in small clinics within their own contingent. They performed the primary care of their own troops. Only when their care exceeded what they could provide did they come to us. We would do some cross training. We would bring some of the other countries' medics over to our emergency room to work with our corpsmen. We were just trying to have some relations with those other contingents, trying to work together. It made for smoother working relationships.

This was the first time any of our Navy nurses or medical people were wearing the blue beret. I did get to bring my beret home. We learned how to wear it. You took the lining out and soaked it in water and then put it on your head and shaped it to your head. We wore camouflage, combat boots, green undershirts and green wool stockings. Anytime one of the contingency people was killed and they were going to be sent home, anyone who was available would line up on the tarmac in uniform in what we would call our dress camouflage. We had a light blue ascot that matched our blue beret and that would be our dress uniform. We would all stand at attention as they loaded the body in its casket on the plane. We were out there one night in the rain. We were all soaked. It didn't matter. When it started to thunder and lightning, we decided we probably better move along as it wasn't safe to be out in that kind of situation.

We had a wonderful morale and recreation department. They had bicycles and movies. They had various activities that kind of kept us going. Trading pins or various trinkets with the other contingents became sort of a hobby while you were over there. Many of us have pins or various devices from many of the other countries. It became sort of a lucrative trade for some folks.

Unfortunately, they made us give most of our uniforms back. I said, "Who is going to want this after I have worn it for six months?" They had my name tag on them, but I guess they would recycle them. I had one that I was able to buy that was my own. Each nation wore their own flag on their sleeve. The Dutch had to cover their emblem. It was very similar to the Croatian flag. They covered it so that when they would go down into Bosnia or Serbia they would not be identified as Croatian.

We had Russians there. If someone had told me that I was going to sit down at night in a dining room and have dinner with the Russians, I would not have believed it. Trying to make food to satisfy the cultural aspects and the likes and dislikes of 26 nations must have been very difficult. We had a dining room where we could all go to eat. It was really kind of neat because you would sit with different people each night. It was cafeteria style and you would just eat whatever was fixed. We used to say that it was savory beef, savory chicken, and savory whatever. We were never quite sure. That got kind of old. The food, quality and quantity were good. It was certainly better than eating MREs. We paid for the food as we went through. It wasn't free, but we got a little extra money in our checks to cover that. The dining room was about a quarter of a mile from our living tents, kind of in the middle of the individual camps.

We had a little post office and a little place where you could cash smaller checks. We could spend our money out in town. We would go out to some little restaurants when we got tired of the savory beef and chicken. Everything was good except for the desserts. I didn't understand that because my grandmother could make the most wonderful strudels. They had flat pastries that were like cardboard. They had very good wine. Sometimes we would get time to go into downtown Zagreb. You could go into a bakery. You could smell the bread baking. The markets were wonderful. You could go to the market and get a loaf of bread for the equivalent of a quarter.

Downtown Zagreb was wonderful, bustling. You could take buses from the Zagreb Airport down into Zagreb, which was maybe five miles away. We wore our civilian clothes any time we went off the base. During orientation, the MWR people arranged for a bus tour of Zagreb. Before we were allowed to go on any kind of liberty, we were given an orientation through the bus tour and a tour guide that told us all about the area. We did some neat things like that to kind of acculturate us. Through that same tour guide, we were able to take some leave time on the weekends and go as small groups to Venice and Budapest. You think you are being deployed. How many people on deployment are able to take some leave time and go to places like Europe? Because opportunities were there and we were not super busy, we could allow people to do that. It kind of kept your sanity. There were people who went to Rome. Germany was a plane ride away. I had the opportunity to take the plane that brought blood to us back to Germany, meet up with some other Navy nurses from Sigonella, Italy, and travel to Prague over one week. Then I took the blood plane back to Zagreb.

The blood issue was something I should talk about. I think when we first got there, they had one freezer that would hold only a few units of blood. When we started taking casualties, particularly land mine casualties, we did not have enough blood. We, as staff, started lining up, a walking blood bank. That can't continue on a regular basis. They were able to procure another freezer and were able to get blood from Germany on a regular basis. I think each group that went in over there improved the system in some way. It wasn't just change for the sake of change. It was, "This is how we can make it better."

Walking from the tent to the bathrooms or showers in the morning or in the middle of the night could be chilly. We soon developed an "I don't care how they see me" attitude. I'm here in my pink bathrobe with my bucket of shampoo. The fire house had a little tent over it, a little fire truck and firemen. I would walk through there because the firemen always had coffee, so you would get your first cup of coffee on the way to the shower. The Seabees tried hard to keep the showers in good shape. Plumbing was difficult. So many times, you would be standing in some water. The showers would be lukewarm or cool. You were really blessed when you got a warm shower. I really can't complain because we always had fresh water. We had six toilets. They were pretty open. It kind of reminded me of the *M*A*S*H* episode with the toilets where the sides, when the wind would blow, would flap up and down. I had visions of Hot Lips when they pulled the sides of the tents up when she was in the shower. I think we had it pretty good compared to a lot of deployments.

For me, it seems like just yesterday since I was in Croatia. In other ways, it seems like a long time ago. Croatia was probably one of the highlights of my career, never thinking that was going to be something that I would be doing. Fortunately, I had my husband back here to take care of nine-year-old Paul. We were just starting to have technology that allowed us to send email with attachments and things. My husband would try to keep me informed about what was going on. You only get a little news. We had CNN on TV over there, but you don't get a lot of hometown news. Wayne would send me excerpts via email. I would have a little email time that I could get on each day. We would have a phone call once a week. The UN would pay for a five-minute phone call for each of us each week. I would call, but then I would have Wayne call me back and we would talk a little longer. That was really something nice that was available for us.

We field tested, for the first time, the video teleconferencing. We would take x-rays, digitalize them and send them back to San Diego for a radiologist to read. We had no radiologist with us. The doctors were pretty adept at reading the x-rays, but just to get the second opinion or collaboration. This was before the age of digital x-rays. We used it for the patients we were taking care of, but the staff could have some issues. We had a staff member who had a history of some kind of a tumor. She started having some problems. They were able to take some x-rays, send them back and have them compared with some previous x-rays. She ended up getting medevacked back to the States. We had a couple of people medevacked back to the States.

The video teleconferencing was used to communicate with Washington. The Navy nurses celebrated their anniversary on May 13. We were able to teleconference on that day with a group of our Navy nurses back in Washington, D.C., from the Bureau of Medicine. We had a cake. They had a cake, so we had a mutual cake cutting. That was a real part of history. I think we took advantage of opportunities like the teleconferencing to break up the routine of our days over there. I don't want to say monotony. You never knew what was going to come through the gate.

I have recollections of a group of new flag officers, who came over to visit the Fleet Hospital. They spent time going through the hospital. They were just on their way out and a jeep was trying to come in through the gate. Well, they didn't seem to have a big urgency, but we had to stop them in order to allow this bus to go out with the VIPs on it. When the jeep came through, I went to the driver. Actually, I think I was standing on the passenger side. Here was this man with fingers just barely hanging on. This was how he was being transported to the MASH. He was French. They had been working, clearing mines. I ran along the jeep to the entrance to the triage area and was able to get him to the emergency room for care. It was just kind of one of those irony things, VIPs visiting and here come the wounded. It was a little surreal.

When you are in theater 60 days you get a medal. It is the UN medal. On the back of the medal it says, "In the service of peace." We had a medal ceremony and lined up on the tarmac. That was one of the special occasions when we wore our blue ascots. They had some of the top-ranking people from some of the contingents to come and pin that medal on us. When we came back to the States, we weren't allowed to wear that United Nations medal. We wore the one that is issued from the United States. It is light blue with the two white stripes on either side. The UN medal was multicolored with green and red. We did receive several other medals, a humanitarian medal and service expedition medal. Probably all told, we got four or five medals. So, if you hadn't ever been deployed, you go over there with two or three medals and come back with four or five. It is just a wonderful memory of the time spent over there. My time in Croatia was one of the highlights of my career.

Coming back and kind of winding down, I returned to my same job at Balboa Medical Center. I retired from that job in 1997. The camaraderie that we shared in the United States Navy Nurse Corps was second to none. The friendships that were formed, the experiences we had, the lessons we learned were all a part of that wonderful experience that I would not trade for any other career.

I think during the early days of my career as the Vietnam war was winding down, I was just too busy learning my job as a Navy nurse and officer to think about the impact of the war on me. The war was still happening "far away." I was in my early 20s and, when not on duty, I enjoyed friends, dating, dancing, and traveling. It was only later in my career that I would identify more with the experiences of the nurses "in country" or on hospital ships and with the "in country Vietnam veterans." While at the University of San Diego getting my bachelor's degree in nursing, part of our clinical experience was in public health, providing services to a cluster of Vietnam refugees. My compassion for their situation grew as I learned more about their lives and their harrowing escapes from Vietnam, losing family members or having to leave family members behind. This experience added another dose of reality to the war. They were another casualty of war.

In the '90s, a play titled *A Piece of My Heart* was written and performed around the country. It was about the experiences of women in Vietnam, including Red Cross workers nicknamed "Donut Dollies," and other servicewomen, including a Navy nurse. I began to identify with some of their experiences, which ran the gamut of emotions from joy to anger to sadness, and "followed" their journey from leaving the States, being in Vietnam, and then coming home. The play triggered similar thoughts and emotions with me of my own experience in a later war in the former Yugoslavia and my participation in a MASH-type unit in Operation Provide Promise. There are common shared experiences because of having served during a wartime, no matter the time served or the area of the conflict. There is a mutual understanding, a true empathy shared with others who have also served "in harm's way." Even to this present day, after being retired for nearly 25 years, as many years as I served in the Navy, the common bond of serving during wartime or in a war zone is a bond like no other and makes us brothers and sisters in arms.

Janet Page Price

I WENT INTO NURSING because I didn't have the dedication necessary to go to medical school. I've always been interested in science. I first thought I wanted to be a veterinarian, but decided I couldn't take being around hurt animals. I'm a real softy with them. I thought about medical school, but by the time I was in high school, I knew I didn't want to spend the next 12 years of my life in school. Given the choice between a nursing diploma program and a college education, I decided to go to college. I have to admit I was more fascinated by my older sister's fun college experiences rather than the quality of the education I'd get. I lucked into my BSN. I had no idea it would make a difference in my career later on down the road.

In 1964, I graduated from Brandywine High School in Wilmington, Delaware. I went on to the University of Rochester in Rochester, New York. Rochester was a pretty good fit. I had four good years there. I spent two years on the main campus, then moved over to the nursing school and lived in their dorm. The dorm was on campus, on the far south side, with the medical center located directly across the street. There was a cemetery and railroad tracks between the main campus and the hospital complex. Going over to the nursing school, you were fairly isolated from the main campus and that made you grow close to your nursing classmates. We lived and went to class in the same building, Helen Wood Hall. The first floor of the nursing building had the offices, classrooms and a big living room area where we could meet and entertain guests. The second floor housed the student dormitory rooms. We did the craziest things. After we finished a test, if we thought it was unfair, or usually just to blow off steam, we would go up to our rooms, turn on our record players and play our music as loud as we wanted. I remember we played *The Mamas & the Papas* a lot, as loud as our record player could go. Sometimes, we keep time beating on the steam pipes. I don't know how the faculty ever put up with us. In addition to learning nursing, we did have a good time.

187

I got involved with the Navy in nursing school. We had two young men in our class who were in the NENEP program, corpsmen going to nursing school courtesy of the Navy. They were great guys a little older than us with experience taking care of patients. They sort of took us under their wing. One of them had a Mustang convertible and would give us rides to the store or town, if we needed something. They got talking about how cool the Navy was, and kept telling us that we really should sign up and become Navy nurses. One day, some of the other students in the class were going to talk to a nurse recruiter, so I decided to go along to see what it was all about. The recruiter was a very friendly, dynamic person and had served on one of the hospital ships. I think it was the USS *Repose*. She did a good job telling us how great the Navy was. I decided to sign up. The Vietnam War was getting to be pretty controversial, but I believed that whether or not the war was right, the guys over there were giving up their lives for their country. I had a way to honor their service, to give something back. I've always thought that sounded sort of corny, but it really was the reason I signed up. The Navy paid for my last year of college. The University of Rochester was pretty expensive at the time, so paid tuition was also another factor, but not the most important. We were enlisted and started getting paid a salary the December before graduation. In addition to our regular graduation ceremony in cap and gown, ROTC held another ceremony where we wore our dress whites. I thought they were pretty snazzy.

I graduated from college in 1968 and thought that I was a "woman of the world." I had a good job and thought I was pretty tough stuff. When I got to Newport, Rhode Island, for Women Officers' School, our recruiter was part of the teaching staff there. Two or three of us from my class saw her and went running up to her and said, "Hi, Pat, how are you?" She turned to us, stern and unsmiling, and said, "It is Lieutenant Commander. From now on, you will address me like that." It was pretty abrupt and really brought me up short. It was the first day of officer training school. They handed us the handbook and told us we were responsible for learning it immediately. We quickly realized it was going to be all business from here on out.

I remember that first night, lying in my rack in this grubby little dormitory, with lights out at ten o'clock. We heard sniffling and quiet crying. There were a lot of sad people. We all wondered if this was what it was really going to be like. They're really hard on you at first, trying to get you squared away and learning the ropes. I remember thinking more than once, "You know, I hope I haven't made a really big mistake."

We all got through it well. We did have some fun along the way while we learned about being women officers in the Navy. We met some guys from the destroyer school who invited us to a couple of parties and showed us a bit of Newport. You quickly started to feel that nobody in the Navy is a stranger because they were friendly and everyone has something in common. It was a sense of family I didn't really appreciate that at the time.

I was in school at Newport for six weeks. I was thinking, recently, about my nephew, who is in Washington working in a congressman's office. He described trying to find a place to live, get food, do the laundry, get enough sleep and all those kinds of things. One of the things

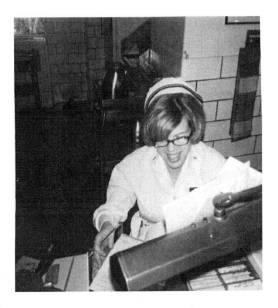

Ensign Janet Page Price provided respect and dignity to her patients in physical and emotional care. She learned to provide quiet dignity to those who were at the end of their lives. Photo by permission.

about the Navy that I really liked was that sense that no matter where you where, you had friends and help. You weren't completely alone.

I went from Women Officers' School to Naval Hospital Portsmouth, Virginia. I was assigned to plastic surgery and urology units. During the day you were responsible for one or two units. Evenings you had four units, which would add two orthopedic units. At night you would be responsible for eight wards. That would add in general and thoracic surgery, and two more orthopedic wards. There was only one nurse for these eight units, but we had good corpsmen helping us. Another factor was that a lot of the patients weren't that sick. You had three or four who had IVs, but most of them were recuperating and didn't require much actual nursing care. At the time it didn't seem that bad. If you think about it though, eight wards with 25 or 30 patients each made me responsible for 240 or 250 patients. That was pretty amazing for someone 21 years old who had just come out of a BSN program and didn't really know all that much. I learned in a hurry.

I was very fortunate to have good teachers at Portsmouth. One of my good friends there was a diploma graduate. I remember very clearly one day at lunch we were finishing up in the cafeteria. She said, "Well,

I've got to get up there and check on my IVs." I asked her what she meant. She said, "Well, you know, check the time; make sure they're running on time." Looking back, that sounds stupid, but it had never dawned on me that you needed to check your IVs hourly, make sure they're on schedule and make sure they stay on time. I was sort of a "set it and forget it" person. I was fortunate that at the end of a shift, they usually came out close. I hadn't been working very long before we had that conversation, thank goodness! The practical things I learned about nursing care, I learned from diploma grads and experienced corpsmen. I didn't learn them in my BSN program. I learned how to put on a good dressing, wrap an amputee's stump, all the hands-on kind of stuff. You were lucky if your patient had something you could learn from, and a ward medical officer who was encouraging and helpful.

I remember working in the ED one night after I had been working for a couple of years. I had never put a foley catheter in a woman since I graduated from college. I had only helped with one as a student. On the hospital units upstairs, the corpsmen would always put the catheters in the men. A woman in the ED needed a catheter. I said to the physician, "I have to tell you, I've never done this before in my life." He just looked up at me and said, "Well, let me draw you a little picture. There's a hole here and a hole there and this is the one you want." That was the way I learned practical things. I had learned a lot of physiology and anatomy in my college program. I am good at figuring things out. I think I have very good analytical skills. I got that from college. I really believe my college education gave me the ability to do that. When I had to do something, I didn't have to do it a lot to figure it out. If somebody showed me what to do, I got it. I look at some of the two-year grads coming out and it seems they can't always put all the pieces together. They may know the "what to do" but not the "why." I believe that's a problem with nursing education today.

I did learn to deal with a lot of different things that they don't teach you about in college. While working in plastic surgery, we had a guy who was having his face rebuilt. Plastic surgery back then was nothing like it is now. We did tube grafts and things that were amazing to me then. He had been shot with an AK-47 in the back of his neck. It had blown away the bottom third of his face. I clearly remember a conversation we had one night. He had saved up some pills and tried to do himself in by taking them all. I never thought my psych skills were very good, but I said, "First of all, you are not always going to look this way." He said, "There's nothing to look forward to. No woman is ever going to want to kiss me." At that point he had this hole where his mouth was supposed to be. I looked at him, "You know, you're right, no woman is going to want to kiss you the way you are now, but you're not always going to be this way. You just have to give these guys time to make you better. You are going to find somebody someday who is going to value you for the person you are, not for the way you look." One day, a few years ago, I found out, through the Navy Nurse Corps Association newsletter, that he was looking for some of the nurses that had taken care of him. I got in touch with him. He was married and had a couple of children and seemed to be doing well. That sort of thing makes it all worthwhile.

While working the urology ward, I called my first code on somebody who was a "no code blue." We had done everything we could medically. This kid had terminal metastatic testicular cancer. I was only 21 years old and it was all in my lap. I just couldn't not call it. I knew he was "no code," but when somebody said he wasn't breathing I just called the code anyway. I was afraid to see someone die. I'll never forget when the doctor came through the door. He said in this cold tone voice, "Who called it?" He was furious. I said very meekly, "I did." He stopped the team and told me to go to his office. I figured I was a dead woman. He came in and very calmly and kindly talked to me. I don't remember exactly what he said, but he did a good job of putting it in perspective. The one thing he did say was, "The only thing we can give this guy now is a good death." That made a lot of sense to me. It was a good lesson for a young nurse to learn. It served me well during the rest of my career. I worked with a lot of different kinds of loss in my work as a trauma nurse. I think anytime you have some sort of personal experience with loss, it makes you better able to deal with someone else's loss in the future. I think facing up to and dealing with loss is a learned thing. Each experience builds on your ability to deal with the next one. This experience was a fairly decent start.

I loved orthopedics. Battlefield injuries create very innovative times in medicine. We did some creative things to manage open fractures before the advent of external fixators. We put people with open fractures in plaster. You would run an IV in one end and a suction catheter in the other end of the cast and run neomycin or some antibiotic through the catheter. Every three or four days when the cast melted away from the irrigation, the patient returned to the OR to change the cast, clean and debride the wound and start over again. We would try things to save limbs that perhaps hadn't been tried or had just been written up in the literature. There was a sense of "What do we have to lose by trying?," and we did save a lot of terribly injured limbs. I remember one young man who had lost a significant amount of his tibia. Standard of care for his injury would have been an amputation. He talked a lot with the doctors and assured them that he was willing to go through whatever was necessary to avoid losing his leg. His surgeon told him he would do what he could. I remember when he was ready for the OR, the surgeon said, "Let's save a leg today!" That fellow eventually did walk out of the hospital with both of his legs.

There were horrendous wounds coming out of Vietnam. They were all dirty. I learned quickly what pseudomonas smelled like. I could walk down the ward and stop next to a rack. I would know that guy had pseudomonas growing in his wounds, even before I saw the classic blue-green color of the drainage on the dressing. That was about the time when gentamycin came out. This drug became our new penicillin. It was the only thing that would get pseudomonas and it was exciting to be able to treat it effectively.

There was a lot of camaraderie on the ortho floors because the guys were there much longer. They were in big open wards where everybody could see and hear what everybody was doing. They really supported each other. As I made rounds through the ortho ward at night it was rarely quiet. We used a lot of traction and as they would hang in traction the chains would jingle and jangle as the guys moved around in their sleep. Sometimes guys would have bad dreams and call out in their sleep. Somebody else in the next rack or down the row would just pound on their bed and tell them it was okay.

The urology ward did a fair number of circumcisions. The ward medical officer and the nurse would make rounds every morning. We would take a chart rack on wheels down the center of the ward. I'd hand him the patient's chart. He would examine the patient and write his orders. I remember, as a very green, young ensign, learning you had to be very careful where you stood. The patients, who were able, would be standing at attention next to their bed for rounds. The doc would say, "Drop your drawers" and the patient would drop his drawers. There were no curtains. I had to make sure I had my back to the patient to give him and me some privacy. That was a lesson quickly learned, with the rest of the patients on the ward standing there watching me for a reaction. I had to know my patients, know who had what medical problems, and where the doctor would be looking, so you knew where to be while the patient was examined. I still believe that if I don't actually need to see the wound, I would do the same thing and try to give the patient some privacy.

The ward medical officer (WMO) was pretty important and how well the unit ran was determined in part by his leadership. I remember one of our doctors was a wonderful WMO. He treated the nurses and corpsmen as colleagues, always taking time to teach us. He would always let us know where he would be and how to reach him. I hated to interrupt them in surgery, so I always appreciated knowing when he'd be back to check on the patients, where he was going and if it would be OK to call him. He had a wonderful way with his patients, too. He was an excellent surgeon. I learned a tremendous amount from him, as well as from several others.

Another physician taught me to listen. He told me one night in the ED, after he had listened to a patient go on and on about her problems, that if you really listened to a patient, they were telling you their diagnosis. They may not be using medical terms, but they are telling you what is wrong. It seems pretty simple, but it made me listen differently to patients and others much more attentively after that. I have benefited from that advice throughout my career. One surgical resident taught me a lot about surgical diagnosis and care during my stint in the ED. One orthopedist encouraged my interest in ortho and was another excellent teacher. I sometimes wonder if the physicians knew how much they taught us every day and how much it was appreciated. It was an exceptionally collegial environment.

Ward nursing was a mix of nursing care and ward management. I remember it was always good to have a bosun's mate on the ward because he was good at getting morning cleaning detail going. They would take the right-side beds into the center, patients and all. He'd get two or three guys in a line and swab down the deck. They'd wait for the floor to dry, move all the beds back and swab down the entire length of the deck. They'd wait for the floor to dry, move all the beds back and swab down the middle. The same procedure was repeated with the left-side beds. They did it every day. This kept them busy and the ward clean. When the nursing supervisor would come through, if your ward was not clean and neat, you'd hear about it in no uncertain terms. They didn't put up with any excuses. The only people we had to do the cleaning were the patients from the convalescent units. Those were guys that didn't need to be in the hospital for care, but weren't ready to go back to full duty. They would be assigned to the wards to help clean or be runners. The nurses didn't go to check the patients on the "C" units. They had first class corpsmen who took care of them, much as they would on ships.

I was on the enlisted units for two years. Then, I went down to the intensive care unit. I remember my first day in ICU being pretty scary. We didn't have a lot of unit orientation at that time. You sort of learned as you went. I remember that only some of the people were on heart monitors. It was before monitors were used everywhere. I learned what a PVC (premature ventricular contraction) was from a change of shift report one day. I was supposed to note if a monitored patient had more than "X" number of PVCs. I asked this other nurse what a PVC was. She said, "Come over here and look at the monitor." Looking at the monitor together, every once in a while, there was this funky wide complex. She said, "That's a PVC. Just listen to the monitor and you'll hear a change in the rhythm." I noted the difference. Honestly, that was how I learned about monitoring. I never had an EKG course. No one I knew did. They just didn't teach EKGs in nursing school. We did have a coronary care unit (CCU) and the heart patients were there. The nurses were trained about cardiac issues and monitoring, but in the surgical ICU, very few patients were monitored and there was no formal training.

There were usually two nurses and four or five corpsmen on a 15-bed intensive care unit. It was the one unit where you had another nurse working with you. I remember we cared for patients on ventilators (more on the job learning/training) and occasionally cared for people following gallbladder surgery. That seems pretty strange by today's standards. I remember one of those patients who died. Postoperatively, she got into all kinds of respiratory problems on a ventilator. She developed complication after complication. It eventually was a pulmonary death. That provided me with another important lesson. I asked the resident, "I don't understand. This woman was like 26 or 27 years old. Why did she die?" He looked at me and said, "Fat kills." She had, indeed, been very obese and probably diabetic. The lesson was that comorbidities matter. It was another one of those life lessons you never forget. To this day, I manage my weight with that in mind.

I didn't stay in the ICU very long, maybe a couple of months. I, then, went down to the emergency department. I worked with two excellent nurses. One of them ran the emergency department. She really showed me the ropes. The other was the supervisor for the outpatient clinics and the ED. She had been stationed in Vietnam at the hospital in Da Nang before it was turned over to the Army. She taught me, probably 90 percent, of what I know about people management. She was sort of this "mother hen" who took us under her wing and made us excellent nurses. She was always professional, practical and an excellent coach and mentor. She was a great supervisor and taught by example. When the ER would be going crazy, she'd come down and ask what I needed. I could ask her to do anything. I could tell her if a patient needed to be cleaned up or a bed pan needed to be emptied. It didn't matter. She never came in and tried to take over. I was the charge nurse and she was just another set of hands. She set a wonderful example and I have always tried to live up to her standards.

One of our chief nurses was also an excellent leader and commanded a great deal of respect from her nurses. She was fair and honest. When she gave you a compliment, you knew it was sincere. Thanks to her, I always wore clean shoes. She came into the ED one morning and looked at my shoes, which were badly scuffed. She promptly sent me to her office to get the shoe polish and do my shoes. I was mortified, especially when I had to explain to her office staff why I was there. I can honestly say that that was the last day I ever wore white shoes that weren't polished and clean. It was more than a lesson in looking professional. It was a lesson in attention to detail I never forgot.

By the time I made lieutenant, I started supervising at night. You got more experience with this job, but you also got more responsibility. The night supervisor had to not only check all the wards and get reports from all the nurses, she also had to go over to another building with the labor deck, nurseries, pediatrics, and psych. I absolutely hated the psych ward where I just felt entirely out of my depth. If it was bleeding, I could fix it. If it was broken, I could splint it. The psych thing, I didn't really understand and couldn't fix. I never felt particularly therapeutic, either. I believe that most of the patients on the psych ward were pretty out of it and I really think I was scared of them. Fortunately, the corpsmen were excellent and helped guide me when needed.

I did have a patient come after me one time, but it wasn't on the psych ward. I really thought he was going to hurt me. He seemed a little crazy. He was a Marine who had lost part of his hand in combat. He wanted some drugs to take with him when he left on leave. I gave him whatever had been ordered, but it wasn't the drug he wanted and he wasn't happy. A lot of the guys got pretty smart about what medicines they were taking. I remember I was standing behind the nurse's desk and he kept asking for more. I told him I wasn't going to give him anything else. He had this big heavy cast on his hand, which he suddenly slammed down on the counter so hard I thought he had broken the counter. He yelled, "I said give it to me!" I was backed up in a corner and there was nowhere to run. Fortunately, my ward medical officer was a big guy and heard the noise. He came out of his office and backed this guy down as the ward corpsmen came running. In addition to profound gratitude, I had a lot of respect for that medical officer. These patients had been taught to kill. Most of them had killed before and acted like they could do it again pretty easily.

I had originally had a two-year obligation, which I fulfilled and "reupped." In 1970, I ended up marrying a Navy corpsman. Fraternization between officers and enlisted was strictly forbidden. I had an opportunity to apply for a billet in Greece. However, I was getting married at this time. I thought it was more important to be married than go to Greece. If I didn't have two really great kids, I would have said I made the wrong choice.

I never advertised the fact that I was married to an enlisted man. In 1972, I was invited to augment from the reserves to the regular Navy. Part of that process was to take a physical. I found, from the physical, that I was pregnant, which was definitely not planned. I figured I would have to get out of the Navy. At that time, you weren't allowed to stay in the military if you were pregnant. It was suggested that I write a letter to the bureau informing them I was pregnant, but that I wanted to augment anyway. It was sort of "you've got nothing to lose" kind of thing. I sent the letter. To my surprise and great pleasure, I was augmented to the regular Navy while I was pregnant. I was told I was among the first active-duty military women to remain on active duty while pregnant, which was an honor. Our son was born March 13, 1973. The day I went home from the hospital with him was also the day my husband was discharged from active duty. He went to college and continued to work at the hospital. I was fortunate that I was allowed to stay in Portsmouth. It was the early '70s. The war in Vietnam was winding down. There were no cross-country transfers. I ended up getting out of the Navy in August 1974, when we moved to Ohio to continue my husband's education. I think that had circumstances been different, I would have enjoyed remaining in the Navy and seeing more of the world.

My Navy experience had great influence on the rest of my career. I had learned how to develop collegial relationships with physicians and other healthcare professionals. When I became a civilian nurse, I was astounded by the restrictions placed on nurses. We had been encouraged to be proactive on our patients' behalf. Navy physicians were open and eager to teach us and encouraged our questions and suggestions. The relationships I dealt with, early in civilian life, were much more hierarchical. Over the years, I saw that change to become more collaborative, especially as physician assistant and nurse practitioner roles evolved. Since I had a BSN, I was able to step into a nursing school faculty position for my first civilian job. It was an evolving diploma to AD program. My understanding of anatomy and physiology, as well as disease pathophysiology, allowed me to integrate and synthesize clinical data and help the students understand the rationale for the care the patients required. My experiences caring for the returning Vietnam warriors engendered a love for trauma nursing. My entire nursing career evolved around developing and managing Level I and II hospital trauma programs. The administrative and interpersonal skills I had learned in the Navy helped me tremendously in my later leadership roles. I have been fortunate to mentor several younger nurses throughout the years and have used experiences with my Navy mentors as a guide.

My time in the Navy also led to an increased sense of patriotism and duty to my country. I was the first person in my family to serve. I am now very proud that our family has many who either served or are serving. My second husband was an Army veteran of 20 years with two tours in Vietnam. My son and son-in-law are in the Army and Air Force National Guard. My grandson is a member of an Air Force ROTC unit in college, with hopes to serve on active duty as a pilot. My husband told the story of his return from his second Vietnam tour to be greeted by a contingent of war protestors who actually spat at the soldiers as they walked by. It was an indelible memory and he never forgave them or the "celebrities" who encouraged them. Today when I see young men and women in uniform, or a veteran with a ball cap or jacket commemorating their service in Vietnam or elsewhere, I make a point of thanking them for serving our country.

I look back on my education and experiences in seven years of Navy service and know that I was more than fortunate to have that foundation. My life and career have been varied and rewarding and I believe I owe much of my success to my Navy years.

Elizabeth Roach

I COME FROM A MILITARY FAMILY. My father was an Army hospital administrator. My grandfather and uncle were both physicians. My grandmother graduated from nursing school in 1916 and worked steadily as a private duty nurse almost until she died in 1989. She always loved working. It gave her independence and her own money. Her sense of herself as an independent wage earner and independent person was something that made a huge impression on me as a teenager.

I didn't really think about nursing until I was a senior in high school. In truth, I hadn't really thought about what I wanted to do with myself. What I really loved to do was read. It was clear that nobody was going to pay me to do that. I heard about the Walter Reed Army Institute of Nursing program through my guidance counselor. I also wanted to be financially independent. I had listened to my grandmother well. The idea of being independent from my family was very appealing. There wasn't a tremendous amount of money. As the oldest child, I felt a real strong obligation to try and get my own education paid for somehow.

The Walter Reed Army Institute of Nursing was started in the mid–60s as a way for the Army to upgrade the educational level of nurses from diploma nurses to baccalaureate nurses. They decided the future of military nursing was degreed nurses. The origin of the Walter Reed program was concurrent with the increasing American involvement in Vietnam. They saw what was coming and decided the way to get a cadre of well-trained nurses dedicated to military service was to actually pay for it. It was a good idea. What I did was apply, wrote a bunch of essays, and had an interview. My grades were always good, so that wasn't a problem. At the time I applied in 1969, there were probably 300–400 applicants. One hundred of us were selected to participate in this program. We would go to any four-year accredited university or college of our choice for the first two years' nursing prerequisites. Then, we would transfer to the University of Maryland at the beginning of our junior year. Our transfer and education were under the aegis of the University of Maryland. We actually lived and worked at the Walter Reed Army Medical Center in Washington, D.C. The faculty members were all military nurses, master's and Ph.D. prepared. There were fifteen or twenty at any given time. We did most of our classes at Walter Reed. Occasionally, we would go over to College Park. All of our clinical work was done at Walter Reed. It was a great education. It was tough leaving home and the University of Kansas, where I did my first two years, and going to Walter Reed. It was extremely competitive. I remember working really hard and being scared a lot of the time. But, at the end of that four-year education we graduated from the University of Maryland with a BSN in nursing. As soon as we passed our nursing boards, we were commissioned in the Army Nurse Corps as active duty first lieutenants. Most of our predecessors had been commissioned second lieutenants.

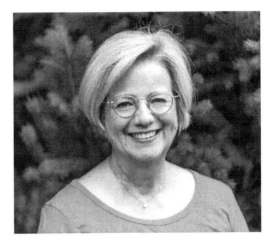

Elizabeth Roach took the lessons learned during her Army experience into her civilian life to provide the best possible care to civilian patients. Photo by permission.

I graduated in 1973. Our graduating class was the first class that didn't go directly to Vietnam from school. I knew that Vietnam was a definite possibility, but I was a military kid. Bra burning was not really in my horizon. In those days, women took off their bras and burned them as an act of defiance to male domination, specifically government male domination. It was the women's movement. It was a really powerful and chaotic time in American history. There was, nationally, a very high anti-war sentiment. I didn't tell too many of my peers at Kansas that I was actually in the Army. I was an E-3 paid inactive reserve until I graduated. The military paid for my tuition, books, and travel. It was a very comfy existence in terms of my financial needs, but interesting emotionally. I was really at odds with almost everyone I knew who profoundly disagreed with the war, even in conservative Kansas. It was a very pivotal time in American history. I felt that I was really at the center of a maelstrom. I was not a rebellious kind of person. I was very patriotic. Service to country and others was very important in our family.

I graduated at a ceremony at College Park, University of Maryland. We walked the stage with everybody else in the college of nursing there, but had another graduation and commissioning ceremony at Walter Reed. We took our boards at College Park, right after graduation. We were told that if we didn't pass boards, we would be scrubbing toilets in some horrible place at Fort Dix, as opposed to some horrible place in Vietnam. Everything is relative. There really wasn't much of a problem passing boards. I think that in all the years that the Walter Reed program ran, only a couple of people actually failed their boards. The program ran from 1964 to 1979.

As I said, I was in the first group not to go to Vietnam. In the following years, as our involvement in Vietnam de-escalated, the need for all these hundreds of nurses dropped off. It just kind of faded out. It was also expensive, but it had some really neat components. For one thing, as a student I not only took care of military and military dependents at Walter Reed, but military wounded that came directly from Vietnam. The most injured came to Walter Reed. There were helicopter pilots and young soldiers of all shapes, forms, and fashions. The ones that I remember the most distinctly and who were really the most formative for me in my experience as a nurse were those young helicopter pilots who had been shot down in 1971 and '72. There were big offensives that took place in Vietnam. We saw the result of that. I remember kids who were amputees and kids who had been trached for months and months at a time.

I remember one young fellow telling me about waking up after this nightmarish existence of being wounded, medevacked and sent back Stateside. He woke up weeks after his initial injury realizing that he was hanging upside down in one of the tilt beds because he had been in a coma. He had been horribly injured. He was an amputee. He had been on a vent for weeks. I will never forget the expression on his face as he told me about that experience. With the next breath, he was telling me, with this incredible swagger, about how fabulous it was to be in the First Infantry Division or the First Air Cavalry. They wore cowboy hats. It was all about the bluster. He was, clearly, so proud of having been one of these forward helicopter pilots, the horrible things they did and this experience in the hospital.

I was 20 years old. It just turned me inside out and upside down. It scared me to death. I knew there was a really good chance I would be going to Vietnam myself. At least I was warned. The experience of older nurses I had talked to indicated that they had gone to Vietnam and had no idea what they were getting into. At least, I had this experience of taking care of these guys and kind of knowing what it might be like.

That it would be hell on earth. You just pick yourself up. You've taken all this money for these four years, have gotten an education and you will do what is asked of you. That was a real family deal. There wasn't much chance of me running off to Canada, which is what others who were trying to avoid the war did. It was frightening.

I mentioned that I was scared. Besides being scared about going to Vietnam, I was insecure. I don't think my emotions about caring for patients were any different from many nursing students. I was frightened about being responsible for another human being, not sure what to do, insecure of my abilities, fear of being unsuccessful and that whole constellation of things that comes with being a student. In an atmosphere of high expectations, all of that is intimidating, to the say least. I was more than a little intimidated by my instructors. Someone with eagles on her soldiers is telling you, "You will do such and such." The commander of this program was a powerful woman. We saw her on a regular basis because she was stationed and worked at Walter Reed. We lived in one building with a house-mother. It was the like the weirdest sorority you have ever seen, or like the old days in the hospital schools of nursing. My grandmother told me about that. I had been in a sorority in Kansas, which was kind of a "fluffy" experience. This was absolutely not "fluffy."

Once I graduated, we had just found out that we would not be going to Vietnam. We found out in the spring of our senior year. We found out what our duty stations would be. Not one of us went to Vietnam. We were told that it was on hold for a year and, after our first year of Stateside duty, we would be going to Vietnam. I was married at the time, so that suited me just fine. I had gotten married right after graduation from nursing school.

I married a man who wasn't military when we started going out. He decided if we were going to be together, that was pretty much what he had to do. He was a junior at Georgetown Medical School. I had met him at Walter Reed. He actually joined the military to do his training, internship and residency because he figured that would maximize our chances of being together. At one point I was an Army daughter, Army officer and Army wife. I also earned more than my husband did for quite some time. My grandmother was all about that. She thought that was fabulous. She was really well ahead of her time.

My first duty station was at DeWitt Army Medical Center at Fort Belvoir, Virginia. The patients I cared for were entirely active duty or retired military. It was quite different from the Walter Reed population. Six months after starting there, I was working on a genitourinary (GU) floor. The chief tools in my arsenal were cans of freeze spray for all the

18-year-olds who were being circumcised. The freeze spray was a spray anesthetic. When these 18-year-olds had erections after being circumcised, it was very painful. The treatment of choice was this can of aerosol freeze spray. For a 21-year-old, even a married, 21-year-old, it was not comfortable.

But working on GU didn't last long. The night nurse in the CCU became ill. I was hauled into the coronary care unit (CCU) one night, completely unprepared. They said, "You are the most recent graduate in this hospital. You are the one that would have had this material the most recently. You are the most qualified to work in the CCU." I may have been scared in nursing school, but there is no kind of scared like a new graduate in a CCU at three in the morning. I was the only nurse. There were corpsmen who were fabulous. The corpsmen were frequently college graduates, sometimes they were premed students. Those guys saved me. I had a couple of books of EKG strips. I would stay late in the morning and pump the cardiologist and the nurse manager for information. I lost 15 pounds because I would go home and vomit. I was so anxious. It was temporary, though. It really opened my eyes to possibilities for myself. I spent another six months in the CCU.

When my husband graduated from medical school, he was assigned to Tripler Army Medical Center in Hawaii for his internship and residency. It is the big multi-service, multi-disciplinary hospital on the hill, a big pink thing. I also received orders to go to Tripler, though I had to ask.

We moved to Honolulu, Hawaii, and lived up above the hospital. For some time, there weren't openings in CCU or ICU. I was working on the gynecology (GYN) floor again. That didn't last long. Within just a few weeks, I was moved. Interestingly, one of the reasons I think I was moved was that they were doing a large number of abortions on GYN, both for dependents and active-duty military. You know, I'm a Catholic kid. It wasn't going to work. I went to my priest and said, "This is something I cannot participate in. I have been asked to assist with a number of them." That was traumatic. Nothing in my military experience was as emotionally traumatic as that. My priest was active-duty military, so he was in a position to make a case. I am really grateful. I had expressed my concern about being involved with the abortions with my superiors, but it felt like they weren't listening. They were doing late term abortions. There were women who had been given more than one abortion, sometimes four or five. They were using abortion as a birth control method. It was completely unacceptable to me. I thought I had made a pretty good case, but nothing happened until I went to my priest and expressed concern. Within a couple of weeks, I was changed to the ICU. I don't know how that change was effected, whether my priest worked on it. I was told that I should pack my stuff and go up to the ICU. I received absolutely no reprisals as a result of my change.

I was moved into the medical ICU. My husband was a surgeon, so I couldn't work in the surgical ICU. But, I was experienced in medical ICU. I worked in the ICU for three years. My original obligation at the end of my education was three years. I extended for a fourth. I was promoted to captain a year after I got to Honolulu and just had a fantastic experience. I worked with wonderful people, both medical and nursing, learned a lot, did a lot.

We were given a tremendous amount of responsibility, whatever we were willing to do within sort of the bounds of reason. I did a blood-gas stick on an astronaut. One of the Soyuz missions had some problems. The American astronauts experienced some gas inhalation on re-entry into the atmosphere. Their capsule dropped into the ocean just a hundred miles from Honolulu. This was probably my second or third year in the ICU at Tripler. I knew something was afoot. I hadn't really been paying attention to the news. I knew something was happening when lots of administrative type nurses started twittering around. Senior physicians were there making sure there were beds open. There was all this concern about confidentiality. I was being asked if I had security clearance. I said, "Security cleared? Wait a minute, I'm a nurse." Then, these three very nice astronauts came directly from the ER. There was a hubbub because there was concern that they had really suffered irreparable lung damage. There were a lot of people working on them at one time. One of the doctors said, "Draw a blood gas on that guy." They thought one of the guys had received the most inhalation. I got my syringe and went over to draw a blood gas, which we did all the time on our other patients. They didn't have indwelling arterial lines unless they had a Swan-Ganz arterial monitor. I stuck him and remember thinking, "Oh, am I nervous about this." We got the blood gas.

At the end of my fourth year in the military, I reflected that my military experience had been interesting and productive. I was working a ton of nights. I was a senior captain more than eight years, counting my enlisted years in school. There were four or five nurses ahead of me. I was not going to be a head nurse because it was such a large unit. The average nurse in that unit was captain in those days. I was getting the tiniest bit burnt out. I was 25 or 26. My husband and I were thinking about starting a family. He was close to the end of his training, so it seemed like a good time to get out. I was also being pressured for a permanent change of station (PCS). In those days changing duty stations was something the military just did. They rotated people frequently. They didn't want people in one duty station too long. I really didn't want to move. My husband was a year behind me with one more year. He was due to be a chief resident in orthopedics that following year. So, the time was right for me to leave the military, which I did, with some trepidation.

We moved to Fort Hood for a couple of years. When the time came for my husband to leave the military, I had—I wouldn't call it a panic attack—but I wept some tears. It was the end of a lifelong relationship with the military, with everything I knew. I knew PXs, military hospitals. I knew how to do everything in the military. What I didn't know was civilian life.

After I got out of the military, my husband encouraged me to take a year off. I had been working really hard. We were hoping to have a baby. As it turned out, I didn't get pregnant until the end of that year. He would come home, and I would say, "I washed the floor today. I did the laundry." Finally, after a couple of weeks, he said, "You don't have to give me a report on what you have done. I don't care. Enjoy yourself." It was really a nice thing.

As I look back on my military experience, I honestly believe that so much of what I know and what I am, as a person, is directly related to my military service. I am extremely proud of having done that at a time when not a lot of people did it willingly. I am proud of having been a member of the Army Nurse Corps with a great tradition and wonderful history. I think that I got my job at Intermountain Donor Services in Salt Lake City, Utah, based on that. About a third of our staff is former military. I work every day with people who view military service as a sacrifice they were willing to make. The fact that I was one of them is something that has really sat well, as time has gone on. It is something we have in common. I have been proud of everything that I did. I don't regret any of it at all.

I think my military experience did affect me spiritually. My experience with the abortion issue was a spiritual issue. I think the concept of service isn't limited to the patriotic sphere. If your mindset is service to others, then nursing and military nursing, in my case, fit perfectly. Nursing is a very spiritual experience. If you let them, you learn from patients all the time. I have vivid memories of working my endless string of night shifts in the ICU in Hawaii, sitting by the bedside of a dying patient and thinking how lucky I was to be there with her. What an intensely personal time that is. Even if you are nothing more than a companion, it is a true gift. My faith has always played a role. What you bring to nursing is your faith and your work ethic. I have been blessed by all of those. I was able to maintain my activity in my church throughout my active duty. That was always a source of comfort. Working in the ICU, people die all of the time. There are horrible things going on. It has always been a source of comfort. It is a great source of comfort to me now.

Stella Ann Ross

I'M ORIGINALLY FROM MONTANA, but I actually went to four different high schools in three different states. My father worked for the American Red Cross in Health and Safety Services. In the early '50s they would transfer him every two years, so I ended up graduating from East High School in Salt Lake City in 1955. I tell friends I became a nurse because I got in the wrong registration line at the University of Utah, which is true (more or less). I wanted to be a physical therapist. Since that's a graduate discipline I needed to get an undergraduate degree first. My high school advisor said I could do it in nursing, which made my mother happy. I was in the program six months before I realized I was in the wrong program. I should have been in Physical Education, then on to a master's in Physical Therapy. I really was in the wrong program, but I liked nursing so much, I didn't want to change.

My first year in the U. of U., I lived at home and took all my classes on campus. We had 44 students in my nursing class the first year. Most of them found chemistry and physics too difficult and changed majors. We finished with 12 in my graduating class.

In my sophomore year, my parents moved back to California and wanted me to transfer. I was tired of changing schools. I had joined a sorority, Phi Mu, moved into the Phi Mu house. The rest of my class moved down to the Salt Lake City/County Hospital. Most of them moved into the nurses' home at the hospital. I stayed on campus and commuted by bus.

At that time, there were three hospitals in Salt Lake City, two private hospitals and Salt Lake City/County, the charity hospital. It was a big cultural shock for me, as I had never been exposed before to the seamier side of life. I got my introduction to drug overdoses and DTs.

All of our nursing classes were at the hospital. We did have classes at night up on the campus. During the day, we spent most of our time on the wards. I didn't realize until later that the U. of U. was one of the best baccalaureate programs in the nation at the time because it involved so much clinical experience. I learned a lot at city/county hospital.

We had two men in our class. The class of 1959 was the first nursing class with male students. One of the guys was a Navy corpsman, still active in the reserve. He came into class all excited with the news that the Navy had just started a Navy Nurse Corps Candidate Program. They would pay for the last year of education: tuition, books, room and board. All you had to do was work for two years after graduation. He wanted to participate so badly, but at that time, the Navy didn't take male nurses. So, he tried to get the rest of us to join. He rounded up four of us and took us up to the recruiter. Of the four of us that applied, I ended up being the only one from my class going into the Navy.

Because the program was so new, I did not have officer candidate status but actually was enlisted as a hospital corpsman (HN or E-3). When I came back to the university as a senior, they wanted me to pay my tuition. The recruiter in San Francisco said, in no uncertain terms, not to pay anything. I wouldn't get reimbursed. I kept telling the university the Navy was going to pay for it, but they didn't believe me. They thought my papers were fake. I finally got a letter saying they were going to drop me from school. I called the recruiter in San Francisco. She flew out and met with the university officials and got that all straightened out. I had a little problem with my sorority when I told them I joined the Navy. Some members acted like I had done something awful and wanted me to leave, but I was the treasurer. I had the checkbook, so I stayed.

After graduation in 1959, I received orders to go home and wait for further instructions. I took my state nursing boards, and went to Berkeley, California, where my parents lived. Many in the Navy still didn't understand about the program. I got a phone call from an angry Navy lieutenant at Treasure Island who couldn't understand why I wasn't standing in front of her desk getting ready to go to work. She didn't realize that I was a Navy Nurse Corps candidate. She thought I was a real Navy corpsman. She told me to report to Treasure Island. When I arrived, she was unhappy that I wasn't in uniform. When I said I didn't have one, she became even more angry. I finally remembered to call my recruiter, a lieutenant commander, who come over from San Francisco and enlightened the lieutenant. I was then commissioned as an ensign in the U.S. Naval Reserve. I still didn't have a uniform.

That changed in September when I went to Officer Candidate School (OCS) in Newport, Rhode Island. I was in the very first nursing class to go there. This was another culture shock. The class before me had gone to St. Albans Naval Hospital. All they did was dress in their nurses' uniforms and take a few classes on how to stand and how to wear uniforms. At Newport we ended up with 60 days of boot camp. We wore gray and white striped seersucker dresses, which were terribly

hard to iron. (We were required to be perfect in
every detail for inspec-
tion.) We only had three
ironing boards for the 60
of us. A few in our group
had been in the Navy as
enlisted personnel. They
taught us about a watch
list. You signed up on the
watch list for the ironing
board of choice and then
went to bed. When it was
your turn, someone would
come and wake you up.
You would get up and iron
your uniform, wake up the
next person, and go back
to bed. Our instructors
didn't know we were doing
that. They were shocked
when we graduated and
told them. But at the time,
we were scared to even say
anything.

I had a roommate
who had been an enlisted
corpsman. She taught me
the finer points of life, like
how to fold my towel in

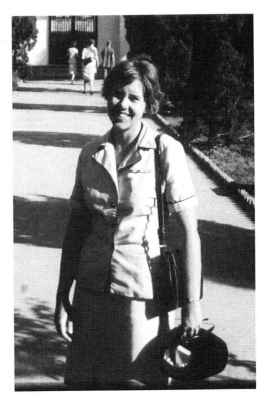

Stella Ann Ross in Vietnam during service
on the USS *Repose*. When faced with obsta-
cles that delayed her ability to fulfill responsibilities, she looked for solutions, saying, "I
have to find a way. I will be late for work."
Photo by permission.

perfect thirds, pin it in place so it would pass inspection and then, care-
fully put it away in a drawer and never use it.

In 1959, from OCS, I went to my first duty station, Naval Hospital
Great Lakes, Illinois. I've never been so cold in my life. It is a lot worse
than Montana. We were in the old hospital which consisted of temporary World War II buildings connected by covered ramps. My ward was
a pneumonia ward with 100 patients. It was a double open-bay ward in
the shape of an H with 50 patients on each side. We kept the sicker
patients on the side with the nursing station, the convalescent patients
on the other side. They were all recruits and we had to keep them until
they were ready to go back to full duty. The pneumonia ramps consisted of four double wards that were down on the other side of a creek

separated from the rest of the hospital. Two wards were active pneumonia, the third, convalescent pneumonia. The fourth was for infectious diseases. We alternated admissions with the other active pneumonia ward. We would admit twenty to thirty patients a day with pneumonia and discharge that many as well. We were always full. On the day we didn't admit, we moved patients. This was really functional nursing.

In school, I was trained in team nursing, which served me well, as often I was the only nurse with two or three hospital corpsmen. But at Great Lakes, we went into full functional nursing mode. On the days we weren't admitting, we would move all the beds. We moved the less sick patients away from the nurse's station in the middle of the ward and put empty beds close to it. We set up each bed with towels and pajamas ready for new admissions. We had every acute patient on vital signs every four hours and cough syrup every four hours. It was written as PRN (as needed) but we didn't have time for that. We had a cart with cough syrup, aspirin, water and everything else we needed and would just go down the row from bed to bed. We took temperatures, passed out aspirin, refilled water bottles, poured cough syrup and moved on to the next patient. When we finished getting around those fifty patients, it was time to start over again. This was a pattern I used years later in Vietnam when I worked the malaria wards.

There were no intensive care units. We had private rooms down at the far end of the ward where we kept the critical patients. We had to set up a special watch to care for them. I learned to have a healthy respect for pneumonia. We had some very sick patients with strep and staph and it makes a difference when you don't have an ICU.

We had antibiotics, but they were not given routinely. The doctors did not like to do rounds at night. Part of the problem was we were so far away from the rest of the hospital. In the winter time, it was really hard to get down there. They really depended on the nurses. I learned to listen to patients' chests. I got to where I could hear rales and detect fluid levels. If we were seeing a pleural effusion, we really had to get orders for antibiotics. If we had a problem, the chief of medicine himself would see our patients. We had so much pneumonia because it was the recruiting center and all these new recruits were living in close quarters. This was before the pneumonia vaccine.

We managed the meals for these patients. The food would come to us by truck in these huge warmer bulk-feeding carts. Part of the job of the nurse and the two corpsmen was to dish out food to all the patients. Of course, we had some bed patients, but all the ambulatory patients would line up with their metal trays at the food cart. We had an old metal dishwasher and convalescent patients were assigned to the scullery crew. They would wash the trays afterwards. I would inspect them. All the convalescent patients had a job since they didn't have anything else to do. They scrubbed the floors or washed the dishes. Some of them even got to go on liberty after I inspected them. I remember this one kid was so proud of his clean white hat. I said, "That is nice." And he proudly said, "Yes, ma'am. I ran it through the dishwasher."

In October 1961, I got orders to Naval Station, Sangley Point, in the Republic of the Philippines. Sangley Point was a little seaplane base on Manila Bay. The squadron (VP-40) was a submarine patrol squadron with big P5M seaplanes. We had a little station hospital consisting of two wards: men's and women's. The women's ward consisted of labor and delivery, nursery, post-partum, and pediatrics all together on the same floor run by one nurse. The four post-partum beds were out on the porch. The one labor bed was right next to the delivery room. On the other side was the nursery with four bassinets. There was also a washer and dryer. There were four Navy nurses: three LTJGs and one lieutenant commander. The lieutenant commander was the senior nurse as well as the nurse anesthetist. We also had four civilian Filipino nurses. The Filipino nurses usually worked the women's ward along with one of the junior Navy nurses. Sometimes one of us would end up having to work it by ourselves. We had hospital corpsmen but no female corpswaves. The Navy didn't send enlisted women overseas at that time. The chief nurse didn't want the corpsmen to be on the women's ward. It was too bad. I could have used the help.

The nurse's job was to take care of the post-partum patients, the labor patients, assist in delivery, take care of the nursery babies, make formula, and wash all the linen after the delivery. Navy nurses can do anything. Usually, we only had one patient and one baby. If we were really busy and I had to go into the delivery room, I would take all the babies out of the nursery and give them to the mothers. We didn't really have "rooming in" at the time, but that is what we needed to do so we could concentrate on the delivery and not on the newborns. One day, the chief nurse walked in and said, "Why is there all this smoke on the ceiling?" I was so busy working I didn't even notice that the clothes dryer was on fire.

The hospital was not air conditioned. The humidity was terrible. We didn't wear hose with our white uniforms. When it rained, the station would flood. We wore rubber flip-flops, and waded through the water to get to the hospital. We put our shoes on after we got to work. All my shoes developed mold in them. When I got back to the States, I had to throw them all away.

We used to stand a duty every other day to be "on call" for

emergencies. In the middle of one night, I got a call that the hospital was sending the ambulance to take me to the crash boat. We had a P.T. boat that would go out every time the seaplanes landed. I was excited to think I was going to a crash but when we got to the dock there was a corpsman holding this huge maternity bag. I thought, "Oh no, we're going over to Manila to pick up a woman in labor." The boat raced across that bay at terrible speeds. I thought, "How am I going to handle a delivery?" Fortunately, she didn't deliver before we got back to the hospital. I'm not a labor nurse. I really don't know labor and delivery.

We also had another boat sometimes used for recreation. A group of us went to Corregidor, which was not that far from Sangley Point. In 1963, the island was just as it had been when the Japanese surrendered. At that time, there was nobody there except for a few Philippine soldiers. If you took gas with you, they would drive you around the island in a jeep. I will never forget going into the tunnels where the Navy retreated during the siege. Off to the side of the main Malinta Tunnel is the hospital tunnel. The patients who were there wrote on the walls. In 1963, you could still see their writings. They wrote their names, their parents' names and phone numbers and messages to their girlfriends. Over the entrance to the tunnel, someone had written, "Remember Me." I have never forgotten that.

I was there 10 months and then I got orders to Naval Hospital, Yokosuka, Japan. At that time, the nurse corps had a system for rotation. Everyone from my OCS class did two years at a Stateside duty station. Then, everybody did a split tour in the Orient. The split tour meant you did one year in some little place like Sangley Point, Taiwan, or Guam and another year at Yokosuka. Our whole class arrived in Yokosuka at the same time. It was one big reunion. This caused terrible headaches for the chief nurse of Yokosuka because everybody was coming and going. I don't know how she stood that.

Yokosuka is south of Yokohama on Tokyo Bay. It was a big Japanese Navy base. They had tunnels going back up into the hill. The hospital was right up against those tunnels. The military command post was back in them, first for Japan and later for the U.S.

I enjoyed Yokosuka. I worked nursery and the women's ward with Japanese nurses. I could always tell when there was a crisis because they would start talking to me in Japanese. I would have to say "show me" to discover the problem. I used to ride the trains and the subways in Tokyo, but I never learned to read or speak Japanese. One of the wonderful things about the subway system in Tokyo, I finally discovered, was that everything is color coded. Even if you can't read it, you can follow the colors and get to the right place. I certainly understand what it is like to be illiterate.

I was there in 1963 when Kennedy was assassinated. We didn't have much communication in those days. I was working nights and we were all listening to the Armed Forces Radio. The announcer suddenly broke in saying, "We're getting a teletype. We can't really read it too well but it's something about the president. We'll let you know when we have more news." So, we hung around the rest of the night and finally they came on and said they had found out the president had been shot and died. That next morning a friend had come up to visit me and we went into Tokyo. Japanese newspapers with pictures of Kennedy were plastered on the walls of buildings. Many Japanese came up and said how sorry they were that President Kennedy had been killed.

In 1964, I was ordered to Naval Hospital, Camp Pendleton, California. This was my first experience with the Marine Corps. Like Great Lakes, the hospital was one of those old ramp buildings with all open bay wards. The open bay wards made it easier to care for patients with a smaller staff. In many ways, the patients took care of each other. I was assigned to an orthopedic ward, another new experience. We had a fire while I was there. Fortunately, it didn't affect any of the patients. The hospital had a center section with an operating room, Navy Exchange, bank and offices. There were two large ramps going out on either side and the wards were attached to the ramps. The fire started at night in the center section when a space heater shorted. It had been left plugged in. The ramps had these huge fire doors that were fastened with weights. When the fire alarm went off the weights dropped, and the doors shut. The only part that burned was the center section. You could see where the fire had gone out the ramps, hit the fire doors and stopped. None of the wards burned. In those days, they didn't call the nurses at home to come in to work in an emergency. The night nurse and the corpsmen moved everyone themselves, beds and all, outside and back in when the fire was over. I didn't even know about it. I drove to work past the burnt-out wing and didn't even notice it was burned. When I got down to my ward, I was kind of upset because the night nurse hadn't made coffee.

I was at Camp Pendleton for two years. While I was there, I applied for graduate school. I was augmented into the regular Navy in 1964 and was accepted for school starting in 1970. Also, the Marines were sent to Vietnam and the Navy brought one of the hospital ships, the USS *Repose* (AH-16), out of mothballs. I immediately volunteered. I thought it would be wonderful to be on a hospital ship. Instead, I got orders to teach at Hospital Corps School, San Diego, California.

I was scared to death. Just to think about getting up in front of other people was intimidating. But the Navy sent me to Instructor Training School. I learned to teach in two months. In the beginning, I could hardly walk up in front of the group and give them my name. By the time we finished, you couldn't shut me up. There were two nurses in the class. Everybody else was enlisted. We all had to practice teaching the rest of the class. I learned how to land a plane at sea, notch a construction stake, and take a globe valve apart. But I flunked the class on double boiler engines. I just could not understand it. When it was my turn, I taught them how to put on sterile gloves. They were just fascinated and walked around, their hands up like they were surgeons. It got me a good grade.

Teaching was hard work. Each class (or company) had 60 student brand new hospital corpsmen-to-be. Each company had two instructors, a senior enlisted hospital corpsman and a nurse corps officer. The senior corpsman taught anatomy, physiology and first aid, and the nurse, patient care. The war really geared up and the classes doubled in size. I ended up with two companies, 60 students in the morning and 60 in the afternoon. We graduated two companies every week. The *Navy Times* would list all the "Killed in Action" and I would compare them with the students I had taught. After a while, I stopped doing that. I just didn't want to know anymore. I was there three years. It was a good experience, but I realized I didn't like being a full-time teacher. One day I looked up and the chief nurse was standing in the door of my classroom. I walked over to her and she said, "You've got orders to Vietnam." I had completely forgotten that I had volunteered, but the Navy hadn't.

I was going to the USS *Repose* (AH-16). Another nurse was going to the other hospital ship, the USS *Sanctuary* (AH-17). Another nurse was going to the hospital at Naval Support Activity (NSA), Da Nang. Three of us at the corps school left at the same time.

My orders said to report for duty on January 23, 1969. My parents were living in an Army base in Japan at the time, as my father still worked for the American Red Cross. I got permission to spend my 30 days' leave in Japan with them. To make travel arrangements, I had to go to the Navy headquarters in Yokosuka, which was still back in those tunnels. No one seemed to know exactly where the ship was, but that she operated out of Da Nang, so they booked me on the flight for Da Nang. My mother suggested I take a footlocker rather than luggage, which was a good idea. Two days before I was due to report aboard, I left from U.S.A.F. Base at Tachikawa, with my footlocker, wearing my dress uniform (wool gabardine) complete with high heels and bucket hat. That was the Navy way. You always traveled and reported aboard in your dress uniform.

The plane landed at U.S. Air Force Base in Kadena, Okinawa. The passenger manager came on board and told me I had to get off, that

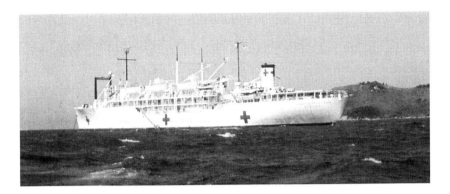

USS *Repose*. Photo taken by Stella Ross and included by permission.

the Navy in Japan had forgotten to book my flight all the way through to Vietnam. I should go over to the officers' quarters and just relax. Another plane would be there in three days. By then, they would have me booked. I said, "Oh, I can't do that. I'll be late for work." He said, "Well, I don't know what you're going to do unless you want to hitch a ride from Naha." Naha was a naval air station at the other end of Okinawa. He called Naha and told me there was a C130 leaving there the next morning. I got a jeep to take me down to Naha and checked in. It was late at night and they told me to go over to the BOQ and get some sleep. The plane would leave at 6:00 a.m.

I don't know why I was in such a hurry to go to Vietnam. A C130 is a cargo plane with four propellers, the military work horse. They load all the cargo in the middle and seats for passengers are just canvas bucket seats that line the outside edges. I got on this plane with another passenger. It took off, but it didn't gain much altitude. The plane circled around, came, and landed again. The pilot got off and gave us a speech about how he had complained about this plane before and was tired of them not fixing it. He said he was never going to get in it again. He left and the other passenger and I just sat there. Somebody came out with a ladder, climbed up on the wing, hammered a little bit, and pretty soon, the pilot came back in and we took off again.

I discovered, by flying this way into Da Nang, that I was landing in the wrong place. People who fly in on the commercial jets land at the main runway with a passenger terminal. For nurses, somebody from the naval hospital comes out and meets them. I ended up landing in Da Nang, on the other side of the river. It was hot and dusty. There I was, with my footlocker and my dress blues. One of the pilots asked me where I was going. I said I was going out to one of the hospital ships. He told me I needed to go over to Camp Tien Sha and check in with the ship locator. The Da Nang complex was huge and had a lot of different camps. Everybody was eager to help me carry my footlocker. They put me in a taxi (a jeep), and we went up to the ferry called the White Elephant, which took me across the river. On the other side of the river was another soldier with a jeep. He loaded me up and took me to Camp Tien Sha.

I got in this line of people standing in front of a booth. The guy in front of me was going to an aircraft carrier, the USS *America*. The ship locator wasn't really sure where the *America* was. So, they had this long conversation about where to find this ship. Then it was my turn. I said I was going to the USS *Repose*. He said, "What is that?" I said, "It a hospital ship." He said, "Oh, I think it's someplace down by Saigon." I said, "No, it's not. It's up here." He said, "Are you sure she isn't down there?" I said, "Yes, she's supposed to be here." He said, "Well, you know, I really don't know where she is."

I was so hot and tired. Finally, I said, "Isn't there a naval hospital here someplace?" He said, "Oh yes, over by Marble Mountain." So, I dropped out of the line and got a taxi (another jeep) to take me to the naval hospital at the naval support activity near Marble Mountain. They dropped me off in front of the nurses' quarters. One of the nurses came out, saw me and went and got the chief nurse. The nurses' quarters were just a string of quonset huts with a sign that said "Da Nang Hilton" but it was air conditioned and they had a refrigerator full of cold beer. Everyone was so nice. The chief nurse said, "You're going to the USS *Repose*?" I said, "Yes, but I don't know where she is." She said, "Oh she's up north and will be down in a couple of days. She goes up for three days and comes down for three days. So just stay here until she comes down."

They put me in the unfinished transient quarters in the back of their complex. It didn't have tile on the floor, just dusty cement and metal bunk beds that were really low to the ground. The chief nurse took me to dinner and then the movies. The movies were held in the officers' club across the street from the nurses' quarters. In the middle of the movie a siren went off, the lights came on and there was absolute silence. Finally, someone yelled, "Condition one." Everybody jumped up and started running out the door. I started running out with them but the chief nurse grabbed my arm and said, "Not that way. Go this way." It seemed it was more dangerous for the women to get in the bunker with the men than to face the enemy. We had to run across the street. The officers' club and the nurses' quarters were close to the perimeter fence and the watchtower had turned its searchlight to face inside the compound. It was a huge, terribly bright light. I was scared to death to go out into that light. Every bone in my body said to go hide somewhere in the dark. But the chief nurse had hold of my arm and the next thing I knew, I was across the street and inside the other building. She told me to go down to my room and get under the bunk. The cement floor was dusty and dirty. I was still in my dress blues but I managed to squeeze under my bunk. There was a flak jacket and a helmet under there, but I didn't know I was supposed to put them on. It was absolutely black because there were no windows. I was lying in the dark and listening to all this gunfire. I think this is when it dawned on me that I was not immortal, that I could die in this place. I thought, "Why didn't I just stay in Okinawa?" It turned out to be a false alarm and the gunfire was all outgoing. Pretty soon, the chief nurse opened the door and yelled "all clear." I got up, dusted off my uniform and tried to ignore my ruined hose. We went back and watched the rest of the movie.

The next morning, I decided I really needed to get out of there and find my ship. I asked the hospital administrative office when the ship was coming. They really didn't know. It wasn't their business to keep track of the *Repose*. Again, I was told to just relax and wait for her. I said, "Well, I can't wait. I'm going to be late for work." But they couldn't help. Then, I saw a helicopter land at the hospital pad and a Navy nurse get off. Somebody said, "Oh, she's from the USS *Repose*." So I went over to speak to her. She was on her way to Hong Kong for leave. She said, "Ross, what are you doing here? The chief nurse is wondering where you are. You are supposed to report for duty." As if I wasn't trying. I said, "When is the ship coming down?" She said, "Well, it's not. It's going to be up North for a while." I said, "How am I supposed to get there?" She said, "Well, you have to take a helicopter." And with that, off she went. I went back to the admin officer, and he said, "I heard she wasn't going to come down. I think they're going to take the mail up tomorrow morning. You can ride up with them." By this time, another nurse had shown up. She was also going to the USS *Repose*. She was also in dress blues.

The next morning, we got our gear and were taken to a helipad, where we were told to wait. A truck showed up and unloaded all this mail while we sat there. It got hotter and hotter. Helicopters came and went and came and went. Pretty soon the truck came back, loaded up the mail and left. I thought that was not a good sign. I went over to a man wearing earphones and said, "Aren't they going to take the mail up to the USS *Repose*?" He said, "Is that where you're trying to go? I'll get somebody to take you up there." Pretty soon, a Marine Corps helicopter landed. He asked the pilot, who said, "Sure, he would take us as soon as he got refueled. He came back, picked us up and flew us up the coast to the USS *Repose*."

I found out later that's what you do. Eventually, I got a list of friendly helicopter squadrons. The Jolly Green Giants were the nicest. You could call them up and say, "I'm a nurse with the USS *Repose*. I need to get up to my ship, which is up north. Do you have any helicopters that are going up north that could give us a ride?" They'd say, "Oh, I don't know. Let me look. Oh yes, I've got one that's going." Of course, they were making a special trip just for you.

The helicopter landed on the ship which was just off the beach from Quang Tri. The chief nurse greeted us at the flight deck and said, "Where have you been? You're late for work." I thought, afterwards, if they had only given us a little checklist and said this is how you do it, it would have been great.

I was still talking to the chief nurse when they announced a hull inspection over the ship's 1 MC (loudspeaker). She said, "Oh, we have to go. We don't want to miss this." I thought, "What? Why do I want to go to a hull inspection?" They announced enlisted off the port side and officers off the starboard. Next thing I knew, I was being ushered down the accommodation ladder into a small boat. As soon as the boat cast off, they started serving cocktails. Alcohol cannot be consumed aboard a U.S. Navy vessel, but off the ship is another matter. The ship's commanding officer (CO) had a supply of "morale alcohol." The ship was going to be on station up north for a long period and this meant that no one could go ashore. He would put small boats over the side and have beer for the enlisted people and cocktails for the officers. So, we sailed around the ship and inspected the hull.

The hospital ships did not do liberty calls. When we did go into port, it was usually only Da Nang. When the *Repose* first went to Vietnam, they used to do port calls and even go to Hong Kong. After TET in 1968, all of that changed. Our mission was to support the Third Marine Division, Northern I Corps (between Da Nang and the DMZ). The two ships were the only tertiary care facilities north of Da Nang. One of the two ships had to be on station at all times. Our northern station was a place called Wunder Beach, due east of Quang Tri. The Marine Corps said they wanted to always look offshore and see a hospital ship sitting there.

The *Repose* and the *Sanctuary* would take turns. One would be on station for three days, be relieved by the other ship and go to Da Nang for three days. On station, we received casualties directly by helicopter from the battlefield. In Da Nang we would unload patients that needed to be medevacked and take on supplies and mail. Usually, about every three months, one of the ships had to go to the Philippines for maintenance. This meant the other ship was on station for two weeks or longer and no one could go ashore. Hence the need for hull inspections.

I was assigned to be the charge nurse for A Deck. In the hospital ships, the decks were lettered A, B, C, D. Below D Deck, they were numbered. The top deck, A Deck, consisted of two malaria wards and one sick officers' ward (SOQ). B Deck was for eye, ENT and orthopedics. C Deck had general and plastic surgery, intensive care (ICU) and convalescent malaria. D Deck had the operating rooms, central sterile supply, and recovery room, which also served as pre-op staging. The lower the deck, the more stable it was as far as motion. The ship was built to handle 700 patients. I think the most we ever reached was 575 patients at one time. We had 30 doctors, 30 nurses and about 200 corpsmen. The hospital ship, being a tertiary care facility, had every specialty including psychiatry, but we only had one doctor for each specialty. However, we also had a couple of general surgeons and a couple of general medical officers.

On A Deck, a couple of junior nurses worked with me. Sometimes, if we were lucky, all three of us would be working, but sometimes only one of us would be working. We rotated eight hour shifts, five days a week. I usually worked days, but not always. The corpsmen worked six days a week. Then, they went to seven days a week. We didn't have that many corpsmen.

The malaria wards had double-decker bunks. Of course, if you had patients on the top bunk, you had to stand on the bottom bunk to take care of them. The Army nurses got to wear fatigues. The Navy said we had to think about the morale of the men. So, the Navy nurses had to be in a white dress and a cap. Not very practical. I would get my cap tangled in the bed springs of the upper bunk. We tried to keep the lower bunks open for new admissions. The two malaria wards alternated admitting days. We would sometimes admit 70 patients at a time, all with very high fevers. We had no place to put them until their beds were ready. I would have dearly loved to set up chairs for them to sit in but there was just no space. They had to sit on the deck, but they were so grateful to be out of the mud. They didn't mind sitting on the deck. We had to get their temps down as soon as possible and the best way was to put them in the shower. The commanding officer (CO) on the ship, a Navy line officer, would get mad because we were using all this fresh water. I understood about water problems on a ship, especially one with old evaporators. But I didn't know what else to do with 70 very sick patients and only two corpsmen.

We worked with standing orders because we just didn't have many doctors. If the surgeons were quite busy, even the medical doctors would be down in the OR holding retractors. The wards might go two or three days without seeing a doctor. We got to be very independent, but we had a lot of support from our doctors. Our standing orders always said, "ambulatory as needed," "diet as tolerated." The nurses made a lot of decisions.

We had FUO (fever of unknown origin) orders for the malaria patients because we didn't know what kind of malaria they had. Every case of malaria was different. If they had Vivax malaria, it was relatively benign and often would go into remission. Falciparum malaria was deadly, if not treated, since it destroyed the red blood cells. The treatments were different, so it really behooved us to get a correct diagnosis right away. Sometimes we could tell by looking at the fever patterns. With Vivax malaria there are a fever spikes every other day and it goes to normal in-between days. Falciparum malaria has a constant high fever which never goes down. However, we really needed a positive blood smear and that meant drawing blood at the right time in the fever cycle. Our corpsmen were really good at getting a positive smear. They knew exactly when to draw the blood. Once we got a diagnosis, we immediately started the patient on the correct treatment. We had standing orders for each diagnosis. We didn't have to wait for a doctor.

We had some deaths from Falciparum malaria because the patients wouldn't take their pills. They thought getting malaria was their cheap ticket out of Vietnam. They thought all they had to do was drink gin and tonic for the rest of their life. They just didn't understand how dangerous it was. Falciparum malaria would cause the smaller blood vessels to clog with the broken pieces of red blood cells. Sometimes it affected the brain first. A patient in the top bunk would start convulsing. After we dragged him down from his bunk and sent him to the ICU, we would find all his pills stuffed into the mattress.

Another complication was kidney failure, also called black water fever. This produces urine that looks like Coca-Cola from all the released hemoglobin. One of our admissions was a Fleet Marine Force (FMF) hospital corpsman. I said to him, "How long have you known that you had malaria?" "Oh," he said "I've had it quite a while." I said, "Why didn't you treat yourself?" He said, "Well, I wanted to be sure you would send me home." However, he had black urine. We started him on Falciparum treatment without even waiting for a positive smear. We scheduled him for the first possible medevac, but he died in the elevator on his way to the flight deck. I was so angry. I thought, as a corpsman, he should have known better.

My other ward on A Deck was SOQ (sick officers' quarters). That was a combination medical-surgical ward. It was a good experience for me, as I got a chance to see serious wounds. We also had those with minor wounds or "dings" who had to stay until they finished their antibiotics. I never saw such a group as those Marine officers who were so nervous about being on a ship. They all wanted to get back into the jungle. One went around and counted all the life jackets. He said, "You know, there aren't enough life jackets for all of the bunks on this ward." I said, "Oh, don't worry about it. We have lots of extras back in the cabinet." Well, that wasn't true. But I wasn't going to tell him that. Our ship didn't have much watertight integrity. A sister ship, USS *Benevolence* (AH-13), sank in 15 minutes during the Korean War. Fortunately, she didn't have any patients aboard, but one Navy nurse died. We knew our ship would probably sink just as quickly, but we just didn't worry about it.

In addition to my regular wards, I stood an on-call duty for the recovery room. The recovery room only had one nurse assigned during the day. In the PM and night, the nurse on duty was a watch stander. We took the watch twice a week. If I had the PM watch, I would go to the recovery room after my AM shift and work a second shift in the recovery room which also served as a pre-op staging area. The *Repose* had an extremely small triage area near the flight deck. If we received a lot of casualties at once, they would have to be triaged outside on the boat deck. The surgeon on duty would do the triage. Incoming patients were put into four different categories: (1) medical, (2) walking wounded, (3) delayed surgery and (4) immediate surgery. Medical patients and walking wounded went directly to the wards. We had standing orders for them. The walking wounded were usually patients that had dirty booby trap injuries. They needed to have their wounds opened, debrided and be on antibiotics for a while. Other than that, they were okay. The debridement was done by the ward senior corpsmen. We didn't do any minor surgery in the OR, because we didn't have enough space. The surgeons didn't have time to do debridement themselves so they taught the senior corpsmen. Delayed surgeries were admitted directly to the surgical wards with standing orders and put on call for when an operating room was available. We only had three ORs and immediate surgeries had priority. For the immediate surgery patients, blood was drawn for type-and-cross and they were immediately sent to x-ray.

It was all assembly line but it was the only way we could deal with a huge number of casualties. In x-ray, they received full-body x-rays, regardless of their injuries, so they wouldn't have to be taken back to x-ray again. At the same time, a couple of doctors would do physicals and take the patient history, if they could. They would take out all the IVs that had been placed in the field, which were usually dirty, and put in central lines. From x-ray, the patients came into the recovery room with a full set of orders. The nurse's job in the recovery room was to do all the IV meds, take care of all the orders, hang the blood which was usually ready by then and supervise the corpsmen. We had huge basins full of soap and sponges and the corpsmen would wash the patients. The doctors would come by and put them on the OR board in the order they would be going to surgery. For patients with multiple injuries, two or three surgeons would operate at the same time. There might be the neurosurgeon at the head, the orthopedic surgeon at the foot and the general surgeon in the middle.

One of the first things I was taught when I went down there was that you did not wait on the doctors. They waited on themselves. They were shown where everything was. If a doctor wanted a trach set, they were to get it and set it up themselves. If someone wanted to put in another IV line, they could do it themselves. My job was to help the corpsmen, do the meds and the blood, which was a full-time job. When the patients came out of the OR, we recovered them and sent them up to the wards. It was a small space, and we were always out of room. If we had a really big push of casualties, they would sometimes operate in the ENT operating room.

Many of our patients were unconscious and identifying them would be a problem. The Marines didn't like to wear their dog tags. They said they made too much noise. If we were lucky, we might find one tied to a bootlace. If not, we would have to give the patient a number, "Unknown American Male Number so-and-so." The number would go on all their paper and bloodwork. Of course, we took fingerprints, but that identification would come much later.

The recovery room was my introduction to multiple trauma. It was a shock since I had been away from clinical nursing during my three years at Hospital Corps School. It was also hard on the doctors. I remember one of the general surgeons sitting in the corner of the recovery room saying, "Why can't I just have a simple appendix or a little gallbladder? Why does everything have to be a multiple trauma?" But, of course, it was. I think, since I worked on the malaria wards, I had a little break. But, for those nurses who worked the operating room, surgical wards and ICU, it was multiple trauma all day, every day. For all of us, there was a feeling of helplessness, as there was only so much we could do.

After my shift in the recovery room, I would get a little sleep and go back to work on my regular shift and ward. The hardest part was working the PM shift on my ward, the night shift in the recovery room and going back to work at 3 PM the next day. It was a grueling schedule, and I would get very tired. Fatigue was a real problem. Before I went to Vietnam, I heard a talk given by a psychiatrist on "The Wounded Healer." He talked about a nurse who pretty much worked herself to death, wouldn't take care of herself, and was devoted to her patients. This behavior, eventually, lead to an early death. I thought he was talking about a Vietnam nurse, but he was talking about Florence Nightingale.

Sometimes, when there were pushes, we would work very long hours. We would work and eat and work and hopefully sleep. I would get so tired I would make some serious mistakes which I still feel guilty about that to this day. We are not supposed to feel that way. I understand about the hierarchy of needs. That the basic needs outweigh higher needs is human nature. But nurses are not supposed to be so human. We are not supposed to put our needs above the needs of our patients. We don't take care of ourselves because we don't think we are allowed to.

Since we were on call to the recovery room, we didn't always have to work if there were no patients, but there were almost always patients. However, sometimes on the night watch, we were able to clear out the recovery room by 3 AM. The previous year, a medevac helicopter trying to land on the *Sanctuary* at night crashed, losing all the patients on board. So now, both ships stopped receiving patients after sunset. Of course, we would always accept a head injury since we were the only place that had a neurosurgeon. The medevac helicopters were directed by a medical regulator, who knew which facility had which capability and which had the biggest backlog operating room space. The medical battalions in the field had orthopedic and general surgeons. They did a lot of emergency surgery during the night and then, they would send their patients to the ship in the morning. During the day, we would get patients directly from the battlefield.

We received most of our casualties when we were at our northern station off Quang Tri. The first thing we did when we returned to Da Nang was to medevac those going on to Guam, Japan, or the States. As soon as we arrived, we had litter patients lined up on the boat deck with their medevac tags, all ready to go. The helicopters would come out and we would offload around 70 or 80 patients at a time. All of the corpsmen not on duty and some convalescent malaria patients would carry litters. The patients would go to the Air Force central staging (CSF) for the large medevac planes. If the ship couldn't get down to Da Nang, as was the case when I reported aboard, we couldn't offload patients and really filled up fast. At one time, we had 500+ patients and had to convert every available space to a ward, even the chapel and the library. We had so many malaria patients that we had to convert the night corpsmen's quarters into another convalescent ward where the patients hot-racked with the night corpsmen. That is, the corpsmen slept in the beds during the day and the patients at night.

I had a patient on the SOQ ward that was going to be medevacked to Yokosuka, Japan. My parents were still in Japan at the time. I gave him my folks' armed forces phone number and asked if he would call them and say he had seen me and that I was OK. We didn't have satellites or computers then, so communication was hard. He did, and my mother was so excited, she drove down to Yokosuka to see him. He said he really wanted to get his wife some nice china, so she went over to the exchange and had a set of fine china sent to his wife. The other patients on his ward all wanted her to shop for them also, but he said, "No, no, she's not a Gray Lady (hospital volunteer). She's *my* nurse's mother." I was really touched when I heard he had said that.

After we finished the medevac, we were sometimes allowed to go ashore. I used to go over to NSA Da Nang and visit my friends. The naval hospital was located near Marble Mountain between the jungle and a Marine Corps air facility. The Viet Cong would fire mortars over the hospital to the Marine base. My friends would spend a lot of time under their bunks during these attacks. I noticed one nurse had a nice comfortable futon mattress, a warm poncho liner, a pillow, a bottle of Scotch and an alarm clock under her bed (along with the required flak jacket and helmet). I said I understood about the Scotch but why the alarm clock? "Well," she said, "I don't want to be late for work." Some of the alerts would be false alarms and last all night. They would be so tired they would just sleep through them.

In August 1969, the Viet Cong deliberately attacked all the hospitals in Da Nang. The ship was up north and the USS *Sanctuary* was in the Philippines. I was off duty and trying to get some sleep. They announced over the 1 MC that the *Repose* was immediately going to Da Nang to offer assistance. I got up, dressed and went to work. But the chief nurse sent me back. She wanted me fresh and ready to work when my shift started at 3 PM. It was hard not being with the action, but she was right. In an emergency, you don't want all your staff starting to work at the same time.

It took the ship a couple of hours to get down to Da Nang, and when we got there, we immediately took on new casualties. We didn't take any patients from the other hospitals, just new casualties so they could recover. Some weeks later, when we were in Da Nang, I went over to visit one of my friends who was on duty when the attack occurred. She was walking from one orthopedic ward to the other. The first round hit the courtyard right in front of her ward. She turned around, walked back into the first ward she had just left and yelled at the patients to get under their beds. She went on to the second ward, and the next round came through the roof of the first ward killing several of her patients. She showed me the beds on that ward. Getting under their bunks was the only protection these patients had but the shrapnel had cut the metal frames as cleanly as a knife cuts butter. Another round went through the roof of the OR and the patient, doctor and corpsman all had been injured. It was thought that this attack was in retaliation for a VC hospital that had been damaged.

The hospital ships always stayed out of mortar ranges. We did have to worry about being mined so we didn't anchor whenever we were up north but just sailed in small circles. In Da Nang we would anchor in the middle of the harbor but the U.S. Coast Guard would come out to the ship and drop percussion grenades alongside the hull forcing up any swimmers that might be trying to plant mines.

I think my most frightening experience in Vietnam (even more frightening than my first night there) was a fire at sea. I was down in the recovery room, which was right at the waterline. I heard the alarms go off and a voice saying, "Fire, fire, fire in the fantail. Set Condition Zebra. All hands man your battle stations." My battle station was right where I was. I was supposed to stay there with my patients. Every instinct in me wanted me to get out of there. But I couldn't. Condition Zebra is where they close and tighten the watertight doors or "dog the hatches." Being on the inside when they close the hatches is pretty frightening. I am not going anywhere. The only thing I could do is hope and pray my shipmates would put out the fire. And they did. I have a whole new understanding of the word "shipmate."

Going to sea is a dangerous business, even in peace time. I had been in the Navy for ten years and thought I really understood it. But going to sea is a whole different world. A lot of tradition, which I used to think was quaint, made perfectly good sense in the context of going to sea. For instance, the ideas of "space and rank." You live in the same place where you work. So, spaces are created to provide as much separation as possible. The officers have their wardroom and the chiefs have their chiefs' mess (dining room). The enlisted people have the mess decks. The captain had his own dining room. Each group, even the captain, is not allowed to visit other off-duty spaces unless invited. This allows each group to get together and talk without worrying about being overheard by a supervisor. It explains why the Navy is so rank conscious. There is no privacy on a ship. I had a friend who was a helicopter pilot. He used to fly out to the ship and visit me. We would continuously walk around the deck while we talked. It was the only way we could have a private conversation. There would be eavesdroppers anyway, but if we kept walking, they could only get pieces of our conversation. The seamen that were out painting the ship would be practically falling off the ladders trying to hear what we were saying. If we went into the officers' wardroom, every doctor on the ship would suddenly be there checking his mail.

We were allowed a week of R&R. My roommate and I went to Bangkok. But the ship was up at our northern station and again transportation was a real problem. We knew if we didn't get down to Da Nang, we would miss our plane to Bangkok. A helicopter from Da Nang landed with a couple of nurses who were coming back from R&R and the pilot kindly took us back with him to Da Nang.

I left Vietnam in January 1970. Fortunately, the ship was in Da Nang. I had my footlocker, as well as a small shipment. Our things were randomly searched for contraband. A friend and I had both gotten a poncho liner, courtesy of some Marine. We weren't supposed to leave for the States with them. I got home with mine, but hers was confiscated. I used it on my bed on the ship because it was so cold with the air conditioning. I still use it. It was so light and warm. The hardest part of leaving was watching the ship sail out of Da Nang without me on it. It was like watching your home leave. I really became a part of that ship. I stayed overnight in Da Nang and got on the plane the next day.

After I left, the Navy started pulling the ships out. The *Repose* was the first to leave and came back shortly after I did. By the end of 1969, the war was really slowing down. When the *Repose* left, the remaining nurses were not allowed to come back with the ship. They had to finish their Vietnam tour and were transferred to NSA Da Nang, or the *Sanctuary*.

Years later, I would always tell other nurses that if they ever had the opportunity to go to sea, they should take it. They would learn so much about the Navy. As for the *Repose*, we still get together at all the reunions. I am also grateful that I got the experience of being in Vietnam. Although emotionally depressing, it was professionally stimulating and served me well for the rest of my Navy career.

I don't believe that I suffered from PTSD, although some of my friends did. I think what helped most of us was the Navy Nurse Corps' policy of not sending new graduates to Vietnam. We had to have been in at least two years and many of us had had other overseas tours. It was easier for us to deal with being away from home and being in a place where there was no privacy. Another thing that helped me was staying in the Navy. I was "career" Navy. At my next duty station, I associated with doctors and other nurses that had been there. We could understand each other and were a support group, even though we didn't know at the time that was what it was. Many other Vietnam nurses, especially Army nurses, got out when their two years were up. They went back to their communities where they had no support. This was even harder for the women than the men because the women were not considered veterans and many were not invited to join any of the veterans' groups.

It was the dedication of the Vietnam Women's Memorial in 1993 that changed all that. I flew back to D.C. for the dedication and one of the things that surprised me was the number of men walking around with badges that said, "Thanks, ladies." It was the first time I really realized that the men felt that way. The male veterans had been gathering at the Vietnam Memorial since it was built in 1984. But this was the first time the women had gone on Veterans Day. We marched down Constitution Avenue and these people were watching us go by. I remember one man who was dressed in a business suit with a briefcase in his hand. We were carrying a banner that said "Navy Nurse Corps." When we walked by, he sat his briefcase down on the ground and came to a full salute. It was the men who were applauding the women, as we marched down the street. I went back to the Vietnam Women's Memorial on the 15th year anniversary on Veteran's Day, 2018. I was wearing my USS *Repose* hat and a man stopped and asked me when I had been on the ship. When I said 1969, he replied, "I was there that year also, only I was a patient." And so, we had to hug.

From Vietnam, I had orders to the University of Washington, Seattle, for graduate school starting in the fall of 1970. Since, it was only January of that year, I would first do a short tour at the Naval Hospital in Bremerton, Washington. It was a small hospital and at first, it was difficult adjusting to the slower pace. Then in August, I moved over to Seattle and started school for my master's degree, courtesy of the Navy. I majored in physiological nursing (formally med-surg). The dean of the school of nursing said to me, "You are not going to finish school. You're too old and you have been out of school too long." It had been over ten years since I received my baccalaureate.

She was right in one sense. The University of Washington program was very physiologically oriented. My first class was advanced med-surg and my basic knowledge was way behind the times. So much had been discovered since I graduated in 1959. So, I had to take advanced physiology with the dental students in order to keep up with my nursing classes. However, I didn't wash out, as the dean had predicted. It was a tough one-year program with a required thesis. I did a clinical thesis on infusion phlebitis, something we really didn't understand in 1970. I spent one month doing nothing but collecting data. I checked IVs twice a day at a local hospital looking for patterns of what caused phlebitis. Even though it was a small study I got some significant results and was able to get my study published later in the *Journal of Nursing Research*. I graduated in 1971 with a master's of nursing.

There were two other Navy nurses in my graduate class and all three of us got orders to Naval Hospital, St. Albans, New York. The director of nursing wanted some master's-prepared nurses to be her supervisors. I wasn't thrilled about that because I didn't want to be a supervisor. I wanted to be a clinical specialist, but my request fell on deaf ears. So, I was the east wing supervisor, which was half the hospital. One of my friends became the west wing supervisor (the other half of the hospital). My area consisted of the coronary care unit (CCU), SOQ, surgery, orthopedics, pediatrics, convalescence and ICU. The third nurse became the charge nurse of ICU, so that was one ward I didn't have to worry about. It was a terrible job. I spent all my time walking from one ward to another and never had time to really learn what anyone was doing.

This was the early '70s. Many of our junior nurses were antiwar. They were not too thrilled with being in the Navy, but they had been candidates, like I was, and were fulfilling their obligations. I was going over one nurse's fitness report with her. She worked in the CCU and I said she had excellent knowledge of cardiology. She looked at me and said, "You don't really know whether I do or not, do you?" I realized that was true. So, I decided to do something about that. I started to spend more time in the CCU. I was really fascinated by the knowledge of physiology and pathology the nurses needed to have. We would send them over to Cornell to be trained, but it was very expensive. Coronary care was very new and the director of nursing really didn't understand why coronary care nurses needed special training. After all, a Navy nurse can do anything. The turnover for these nurses was very fast. When their two years were up, they would get out of the Navy. When Cornell announced that they were going to raise the fees from $100 to $500, I thought that was my opportunity. One thing I learned about the Navy is when you see an opportunity, you better grab it.

I told the director of nursing that if she sent me to coronary care training, I would return and train everyone else since I used to teach and I was career Navy. It would save the command a lot of money and she agreed. They sent me to St. Vincent's Hospital on Staten Island because it was cheaper than Cornell but it was still an excellent program. It was four weeks: three academic and one clinical. Then I came back and worked in the CCU and someone else became the east wing supervisor. I was technically the CCU supervisor and continued to report directly to the director of nursing. I set up a one-week course, eight hours a day, with lesson plans and training aids. I covered everything from pathophysiology to coronary risk factors with an emphasis on cardiac arrhythmias. It was pretty bare bones instruction, but I was able to train the nurses and the corpsmen. I loved that I was doing both the work and the teaching. I had a lot of autonomy. It was like being back in Vietnam.

We worked with protocols. We were expected to diagnose and treat arrhythmias, according to the protocols, without waiting for a doctor. The cardiologist told me that my knowledge was that of a medical resident level and I should not let doctors, who were not cardiologists, tell me what to do, especially when it came to myocardial infarction and cardiac arrhythmias. Sometimes, they would put medical students in my class to learn about arrhythmias since it was not something that they taught in medical school.

I was there a couple of years. In January 1974, the Navy decided to close the hospital at St. Alban's. I got orders to the Naval Medical Command, Camp Lejeune, North Carolina, and was told they needed a CCU supervisor. However, those orders were delayed due to a controversary over St. Alban's closing. By the time I finally got to Camp Lejeune, I had been promoted to full commander. The chief nurse asked me where I wanted to work. I told her I wanted to work in CCU. She said that their unit was a combined ICU/CCU unit and because my orders had been held up, she had put somebody else in that position. Besides, I was full commander and should be a supervisor. She said I should take some time and look the hospital over. While I was doing that, I went to the command Welcome Aboard party and ran into the cardiologist. He saw I was new and said, "What do you do?" I said, "I'm a coronary care nurse" and he said, "Oh, I feel like giving you a hug and a kiss right now." I said, "What?" He said, "Well, we don't have any," and I said, "But you have a CCU?" He said, "Yes, but we don't have any CCU nurses."

The next day, I went up to the ICU/CCU and discovered he was right. The CCU consisted of a four-bed glassed-in section at the end of a big open bay ward that was the ICU. The charge nurse, who had taken the supervisor position, was an ICU nurse but knew nothing about coronary care. The junior nurses assigned to the CCU had never been trained. They were scared to death because they knew they didn't know what they were doing. However, they got no sympathy from either the ICU charge nurse or even the chief nurse because neither understood why coronary care was different. It was another case of "a Navy nurse can do anything." First, I thought, "Why didn't this doctor train these nurses himself if he's so upset about it?" Well, he didn't like to teach. Instead, he put a monitor in his office. If he had an unstable patient, he would go to his office and spend the night watching the monitor himself, instead of trusting the nurses.

I told the chief nurse that I wanted to work CCU. She didn't say no. I think by this time the cardiologist and the chief of medicine had gotten to her. But she did say she thought it would ruin my career going back to being a charge nurse and I would never make captain. I know she was looking out for my career and my interests, but for me there was no choice. I thought, "I have the ability and knowledge to train those nurses. If I don't do that, I will never be able to live with myself." I got both the ICU as well as the CCU, since they were a combined unit. Then I told her I wanted to set up classes like I had at St. Alban's. I still had all the lesson plans and training aids. But she said, "Oh, no. That's a luxury only civilian hospitals can afford." It wasn't that it cost money. She didn't want to spare the time and again, didn't think any training was necessary.

So, I taught in the evening after she left for the day. I set the class to run from 5:00 to 6:00 p.m. in the cardio-pulmonary lab, kind of hidden from everything but close to the ICU. The night nurses and corpsmen would come in at 5:00 p.m. and the day people would stay after work. The evening shift would come during their dinner hour. Since I could only teach one hour a day, it took a long time to finish the course. But I did get everyone through. I don't think the chief nurse ever knew about it or at least she never said anything.

Since I was also responsible for the ICU, I had to learn about the full gamut of critical care, including patients on ventilators. That was a real challenge. I studied hard and passed the exam to be certified as a critical care RN. I was told that I was the first Navy nurse to achieve that certification.

One of the nice things about the Navy is that nothing ever stays the same. Pretty soon the chief nurse left and was replaced by one who was very clinically and educationally oriented. The first thing she said to me, when she arrived, was, "Well, are you teaching a class?" I was there for four and a half years and loved every minute of it.

Navy nurses have a custom of sending a command Christmas card to the nurses at other duty stations. In 1977, a Christmas card arrived with a nurse sitting on a camel in front of a pyramid. Somebody said that was "our nurse in Cairo." She was stationed at the Navy Medical Research Unit #3 (NAMRU-3) in Cairo, Egypt (a one nurse billet or position), and was the first nurse to go there. I thought that looked exciting, so I put in a request card and was almost immediately contacted by my detailer. She wanted to know if I had really requested that, and if so, was I willing to stay at Camp Lejeune until fall 1978 when the Cairo billet would be available. Of course I was.

I got to Egypt in September 1978. The country was still at war with

Israel, although they had a ceasefire. There were soldiers everywhere and you didn't dare take pictures. Sadat had made the Russian military leave and vowed to never again allow foreign military in Egypt. We were allowed to stay because we were sponsored by the Ministry of Health and performing a humanitarian mission. There was no American base. The unit was tucked into the corner of the local fever hospital and maintained a low profile. We didn't fly the American flag or wear military uniforms. We came under the auspices of the U.S. Embassy, carried embassy ID cards and had embassy license plates on our cars. We all lived on the economy.

The Navy has research units around the world studying infectious diseases. NAMRU-3 has been in Cairo in some form since 1947 when it took over from the British Typhus Commission. They had three areas of research: laboratory research, an animal section and clinical investigation, where I worked in clinical support. We had a ward for Egyptian patients set up on the American model by the first Navy nurse to be assigned. There were four Egyptian nurses, one male and three female, all trained by the French and British. They spoke and charted in English. We also had male nursing attendants, who also spoke English. My job was to supervise them. Their clinical experience was different than American nurses. Much had to do with the culture. Women of good reputation did not provide direct patient care. If any of the Americans became sick, I took care of them myself. Even so, the French and British trained nurses were far better than most Egyptian nurses.

We were primarily studying schistosomiasis, which is caused by parasites who live in freshwater snails. If untreated, it can cause serious and even fatal intestinal and kidney disease. Like any infectious disease, it has major implications for military readiness. We were studying the effectiveness of different medications. Our patients came to us for treatment, and we treated everyone. If they fit our research protocol, we admitted them to the ward. If not, we treated them as outpatients. If they were very ill but did not fit the protocol, we admitted them and treated them out-of-study. We never turned anyone away without treating them.

We also had a meningitis project in the fever hospital next door. We saw patients with encephalitis and meningitis due to tuberculosis but mostly our patients had Rift Valley Fever and that was the focus of our research. Rift Valley Fever (RVF) is caused by a virus which primarily infects animals, but can infect humans. It was first identified in 1931, during an epidemic among sheep on a farm in the Great Rift Valley of Kenya. An explosive outbreak occurred in Egypt in 1977, the year before I got to Cairo. It has different clinical features. In the mild form, it is like dengue, also called Break Bone Fever, with a high fever and severe pain (as if every bone was breaking). Then it often subsides with no sequalae. The hemorrhagic form is similar to Ebola and Lassa fevers with massive bleeding and is 50 percent fatal. There is also an ocular version with macular degeneration and permanent loss of vision. Meningoencephalitis with residual neurological deficit can occur. I saw one patient with macular degeneration and one of our Americans had the high fever which subsided. However, the meningitis ward was full of RVF patients who were no longer acutely ill but suffering from the aftermath with partial paralysis. Some had been in a coma for over a year.

In 1977, when Rift Valley Fever first burst on the scene in Egypt, NAMRU was actively involved in the research and eventual identification of the virus. As luck would have it, it had been studied by the U.S. Army back in the '50s as a possible bio-terrorism agent. They had developed a vaccine, which was still available. NAMRU started vaccinating as many Americans and Egyptians as they could. When I got there in September 1978, the epidemic was still running its course. I was also vaccinated. The unit was still actively studying RVF and in the next year, discovered it was carried by a mosquito.

Going over to the fever hospital was like walking back in time 100 years. The wards were really run down. However, to prevent our research from being compromised, the Navy had renovated the ward we used by painting it and bringing the sanitation up to American standards. Still, in regard to nursing care, it was quite the cultural change. The nurses only spoke Arabic. I studied Arabic for the entire two years and got to be fairly comfortable with the language. I could understand what was going on around me, but I never was a fluent speaker. I learned the alphabet so I could read street signs and find doctors' offices. Again, it was another country where I knew what it was like to be illiterate.

The nurses didn't do direct patient care because of their culture. In that culture, a woman doesn't touch a man not related to her. So, every patient had to have a family member at the bedside to be the caregiver. The nurse supervised the family and passed out medications. Sometimes, the patients would need intravenous infusions (IVs). We brought the IVs from NAMRU, and the Navy pharmacy technician would make them up for us. The nurses didn't have time to watch the IVs, so I would teach the patients' families how to take care of them. Even though some of the caregivers didn't speak English, they were very smart and I got to be really good at sign language.

Mostly, what I did would be considered rehabilitation. I worked with the patients recovering from comas who had suffered contractures or were partially paralyzed. They needed to be able to walk and care for themselves. Everything was very primitive. We didn't have much modern equipment. I didn't really accomplish a lot but it was very gratifying.

However, I learned a lot. Egypt was a wonderful experience. When I got the orders to go over there, the girl I relieved said to me, "If you don't mind dust and flies and you like art and history, you'll be in fat-city. If it's the other way around, you'll be miserable." I love art and history. I grew up camping in Montana, so I didn't mind dust and flies. I was entitled to a household shipment, but she told me not to bring anything I couldn't walk away from. So, I took my car and some furniture but no family heirlooms or anything of value. I had my own apartment. The Navy rented two buildings for the single members, one for enlisted and another for officers. There were three of us in our building: an engineer, the virologist and me. The electricity was 220 and very unreliable. We had power outages and often went without water. I learned to keep candles handy and to always store water. We had canteen privileges at the American Embassy and could buy liquor and a few other odds-and-ends. I would save the liquor bottles and fill them up with water. The first Arabic I learned was "mafeesh maya" (there's no water). The other two guys and I went in together and hired a cook. He fixed breakfast and dinner six days a week. He also did the shopping, which was a daily chore. There were no supermarkets, and nothing was refrigerated. I had a tiny refrigerator, but it didn't hold much.

I was living alone and sometimes this proved interesting. In the Egyptian culture, women did not have their own apartments. A woman should have a male protector: husband, father or brother. Otherwise, she is not a woman of good reputation. One day my washing machine wasn't working well. I called an Egyptian repairman and when he came, he said, "Oh, nice apartment. Where's your husband?" I said, "I'm not married." And then, "Where's your father?" I said, "He's back in the States." Then he said, "Oh, you live alone?" I said, "No, I have two brothers next door. Do you want to meet them?" He said, "No, that's okay" and went to work on the washing machine. There were times I would have to actually knock on the engineer's door and he would come to the door and show his face. The guys were really nice about that. Because I was an American, I did have some freedom but I still had to be careful to follow the social rules. I had my car and could drive by myself during the day, but I didn't go out at night without an escort.

In March 1979, the Camp David Peace Treaty was signed. Suddenly everything was different. We knew that President Carter was going to come and visit, but we really didn't know when. A Navy commander visiting the embassy came to see me and wanted to know what I thought of the local hospitals. "Why do you want to know?" I asked. He said, "Well, I can't tell you." So, I said, "Well, if I was expecting a very important member of the U.S. government to visit, I would have an aircraft carrier with a surgical team aboard sitting off the coast at Alexandria." He said, "Thank you very much," and got up and left. I found out later that that is exactly what they did for the president's visit.

It was all a big secret as to when he was actually going to arrive. However, I heard that the airport would be closed between 2:00 and 4:00 on Sunday. The airport road was only a couple of blocks from my apartment, so I walked over there at 2:00 PM that Sunday. The street lights were adorned with little American and Egyptian flags. That was the first time I had ever seen an American flag flying in Egypt any place except the Embassy. There were already people gathering along the street. I sat there for maybe a couple of hours. Pretty soon the motorcade came along. I took a picture of presidents Sadat and Carter together in the lead car.

The next big event occurred in November of that year when the Iranians took over the U.S. Embassy in Tehran. We didn't have English language TV and our telephones didn't work so I didn't know anything about it until I drove up to our front gate. I knew something was up when I saw the sleepy little policeman at the gate had been replaced by a rather alert Army soldier with an automatic weapon. The unit could communicate with the Embassy via a secure landline the Embassy had placed. I got the news when I got inside. The Egyptian government was really worried that the same thing was going to happen there with the Islamic fundamentalists. They took immediate steps to protect the Embassy. Nothing ever happened, but there were a lot of routine changes. You could tell the security had increased. We did work on an evacuation plan and decided that it wouldn't work unless we had the help and support of our Egyptian coworkers. We were paid in Egyptian pounds but our unit did have an evacuation supply of U.S. currency if we needed it. Fortunately, we didn't. The only time the unit had ever been evacuated was to Naples, Italy, during the Yom Kippur War in 1967. During the 1973 war, they stayed in place.

I left Egypt in the fall of 1980 and went to the Naval Regional Medical Center at Portsmouth, Virginia. I was a captain. Director of continuing education was the only billet that was available. I soon realized education was not my interest. If I could not go back to the clinical, I might as well go into nursing administration. I asked the chief nurse if I could replace the assistant chief nurse, who was medically retiring. She agreed and taught me so much. She taught me how to deal with politics, how not to sweat the small stuff and to pick your battles. It was great.

I was supposed to be there three years, but in March 1983 I got orders to the office of the chief of naval operations in Washington, D.C. This was a brand-new position which I hadn't requested. Specifically, I was on the staff of the Navy surgeon general (OP-093) who came under the vice chief of naval operations. I was a quality assurance analyst. There were four of us in the quality assurance section: doctor, dentist, medical service officer and me, a nurse. Anytime there was a complaint regarding military medicine, it would come to our office. One of us would be responsible for investigating and writing the response. I always got the ones involving nurses.

There was a nurse who complained that she had to work nights at Naval Hospital, Bethesda. She sent that letter to her senator. He sent a letter over to the Navy department with a long dissertation about circadian rhythms and how rotating shifts was not a good idea. I had to respond to this for the surgeon general's signature. I wrote that even though I agree with him, the Navy did not pay a differential for the evening or night shift, and therefore everybody had to take their turn rotating shifts. The surgeon general signed it and I never heard another word about it.

For some reason, I also got all the tasks relating to decedent affairs. I had to explain to a grieving man why the Navy could not retrieve his brother's remains from a World War II crash on a Canadian mountain. I had to explain why the Navy shot holes in a casket because it didn't sink during a sea burial. I responded about why a helicopter pilot's ashes could not be thrown out of a helicopter. Each time I had to investigate the case meant several trips over to the Pentagon. We didn't have email in those days, so I did a lot of going back and forth. In the case of the helicopter pilot's ashes, I was reminded that the ashes would be pulled into the updraft of the main rotor and might foul them. I was embarrassed that I didn't remember that from all the times I had flown in helicopters in Vietnam.

I was the Navy Nurse Corps planning officer. I wrote the instructions for nurses coming into the Navy. The secretary of the Navy wanted all of the procurement instructions for the medical department to be identical. Easier said than done since nurses had to be different. At that time (1983), we were still taking nurses who were three-year graduates from hospital programs. We didn't want associate degree nurses since we thought the two-year program didn't prepare them for the leadership role of a naval officer. The rest of the Navy required a baccalaureate degree for an officer, but the nurse corps didn't think we could fill our numbers with just baccalaureate nurses. The war-fighting side of the Navy (line officers) couldn't understand why nurses were different. The Nurse Corps couldn't understand why the line officers cared.

I was right in the middle. I worked with a line officer from the secretary of the Navy's office. We argued over every word in that instruction. The Nurse Corps wanted a school's curriculum defined by a certain number of hours that would admit the three-year graduates but not the two-year graduates. The line officer didn't understand that at all. Then I would go back to the director of the Nurse Corps. Her assistant would say, "Just tell them that's the way we do it." I said, "I can't tell the secretary of the Navy that. I have to give good reason for the way we do it."

It took two years working on this instruction before I got both sides to agree with the wording. When the secretary of the Navy signed that instruction, I broke out the champagne. The director of the Nurse Corps presented me with a framed copy of the instruction with "Congratulations for a job well done" written on it. That is one of my prize possessions.

I was also involved in projects concerning Navy hospital corpsmen. The surgeon general decided he wanted to replace the independent duty corpsmen on attack submarines with Navy physician's assistants. From a medical viewpoint, that makes excellent sense. Attack submarines do not carry doctors and although the submarine independent duty corpsmen are very well trained, a physician's assistant would have further education with an associate degree. That was easier said than done, as I discovered very quickly when I went over to the Pentagon to talk to the submarine community. They were just horrified that I even suggested it. It didn't matter that we were offering them better medical care, we would be upsetting the whole rank structure on the submarine. An independent duty corpsman is an enlisted man, but a physician's assistant is a warrant officer. I had visited an attack submarine when I was in Portsmouth, so I knew how crowded they were. The corpsmen bunked with the torpedo tubes as do the rest of the enlisted, but the officers had staterooms. There weren't any extra staterooms, and the warrant officer certainly wasn't going to bunk with the captain. Where was he going to eat? The officers' wardroom was too small for even one more chair. Since I had spent a year on a ship, I did understand their concerns. Now I had to convince the surgeon general. I was very nervous about going back to my boss and saying his idea wasn't going to work. So I put together a briefing book with all the pros and cons. I worked hard on this and when I presented it to him with my recommendation that we not take action, he just sighed and said, "OK."

In 1985, at the end of my two-year tour, I was just beginning to understand the job of being a staffer and I probably should have extended for another year. I wanted to get back to a hospital. I received orders to Naval Regional Medical Center, Memphis, Tennessee, where

I was the director of nursing. I felt that it was an opportunity to put all of what I had learned throughout my Navy career to good use. I particularly enjoyed working with the junior nurses and helping them with their careers.

I stayed in Memphis for five years and retired from the Navy in 1990. I had reached statutory retirement and had to leave active duty, but I was ready. I had a very nice retirement ceremony. Since I never got married, my ceremony was my big event. A former director of the Navy Nurse Corps was the guest speaker. My parents were there, and I had lots of out-of-town guests and friends.

I started my Navy career with the requirement to serve for only two years and ended up serving 31. Along the way, I had a lot of adventures and experiences that many nurses only dream about, although in most cases, it was just a matter of being in the right place at the right time. Each experience seemed to prepare me for the next one coming around the corner. I do appreciate how fortunate I am.

In looking back at my year in Vietnam, I have to say it was the most significant year of my career. What I learned affected me both personally and professionally for the rest of my life. On a personal note, I learned a lot about myself and not all of it was good. I have a lot of guilt about that. It was hard work. Sometimes, I worked to the point of exhaustion. There were times when I was so tired, all I could think of was getting some rest. I never actually put my needs ahead of those of my patients, but there were times I wanted to and I still feel terrible about that. Nurses are not supposed to be so human.

When I first visited the Vietnam Memorial, I thought I would pay my respects to those of my patients who had died, but I was shocked to realize that I didn't remember any of their names. I could remember their injuries, how it happened, even when and where, but not their names. I know that is probably a defense mechanism and may be why I really didn't suffer from any PTSD afterwards. But still, it's terrible not to remember someone's name.

However, I also learned a lot professionally. I learned fast about combat casualty care. I had been teaching at basic corps school for three years and had not seen the injuries caused by high velocity weapons. The first evening I worked in the Recovery room/pre-op staging area, I went to help a corpsman clean a patient covered with mud. I lifted up his foot to clean his leg and the foot came apart in my hand. There was no leg left. It was quite a shock, but I didn't have time to think about it as there was too much to do.

I learned to be better organized, to think critically, to be confident in my own knowledge and abilities. We had a lot of autonomy and were treated by our doctors with a great deal of respect. We learned to diagnose and treat within certain guidelines. It was all very stimulating and furthered my professional growth.

I also learned a lot about the Navy. It is a sea-going service and to be a true member of the Navy, one really needs to go to sea. It's a dangerous business, even in peacetime. I learned how easy it is for ships to sink. Once I faced the realization that I was not immortal, I didn't have to worry about it anymore.

I also learned the true meaning of the word "shipmate." It's often applied to anyone you ever knew, but a real shipmate is one you served with on a real ship. One of my *Repose* shipmates had to be medically retired due to ovarian cancer. I wrote this poem for her at her retirement.

SHIPMATES

Shipmates
are people
        you work with
        live with
        fight with
        get drunk with.

Shipmates
are people
        you share things with.

things like—danger
        fear
        comfort
        safety
        confinement
        loneliness
        companionship
        liberty
        bad times
        good times

Shipmates
are people
        you never forget.

USS *Repose* (AH-16)
1969

Index